Understanding the Patellofemoral Joint: From Instability to Arthroplasty

Editor

ALEXANDER K. MEININGER

CLINICS IN
SPORTS MEDICINE

www.sportsmed.theclinics.com

Consulting Editor
MARK D. MILLER

July 2014 • Volume 33 • Number 3

ELSEVIER

1600 John F. Kennedy Boulevard • Suite 1800 • Philadelphia, Pennsylvania, 19103-2899

http://www.theclinics.com

CLINICS IN SPORTS MEDICINE Volume 33, Number 3
July 2014 ISSN 0278-5919, ISBN-13: 978-0-323-32075-7

Editor: Jennifer Flynn-Briggs
Developmental Editor: Donald Mumford

Clinics in Sports Medicine (ISSN 0278-5919) is published quarterly by Elsevier Inc., 360 Park Avenue South, New York, NY 10010-1710. Months of issue are January, April, July, and October. Business and Editorial Offices: 1600 John F. Kennedy Blvd., Ste. 1800, Philadelphia, PA 19103-2899. Customer Service Office: 3251 Riverport Lane, Maryland Heights, MO 63043. Periodicals postage paid at New York, NY and additional mailing offices. Subscription prices are $340.00 per year (US individuals), $540.00 per year (US institutions), $165.00 per year (US students), $385.00 per year (Canadian individuals), $666.00 per year (Canadian institutions), $235.00 (Canadian students), $470.00 per year (foreign individuals), $666.00 per year (foreign institutions), and $235.00 per year (foreign students). Foreign air speed delivery is included in all *Clinics* subscription prices. All prices are subject to change without notice. **POSTMASTER:** Send address changes to *Clinics in Sports Medicine*, Elsevier Health Sciences Division, Subscription Customer Service, 3251 Riverport Lane, Maryland Heights, MO 63043. Customer Service (orders, claims, online, change of address): Elsevier Health Sciences Division, Subscription Customer Service, 3251 Riverport Lane, Maryland Heights, MO 63043. Tel: 1-800-654-2452 (U.S. and Canada); 314-447-8871 (outside U.S. and Canada). Fax: 314-447-8029. E-mail: journalscustomerservice-usa@elsevier.com (for print support); journalsonlinesupport-usa@elsevier.com (for online support).

Reprints. For copies of 100 or more of articles in this publication, please contact the Commercial Reprints Department, Elsevier Inc., 360 Park Avenue South, New York, NY 10010-1710. Tel.: 212-633-3874; Fax: 212-633-3820; E-mail: reprints@elsevier.com.

Clinics in Sports Medicine is covered in *MEDLINE/PubMed (Index Medicus) Current Contents/Clinical Medicine, Excerpta Medica,* and *ISI/Biomed.*

Contributors

CONSULTING EDITOR

MARK D. MILLER, MD
S. Ward Casscells Professor; Head, Division of Sports Medicine, Department of Orthopaedic Surgery, University of Virginia; Team Physician, James Madison University, Charlottesville, Virginia

EDITOR

ALEXANDER K. MEININGER, MD
Orthopaedic Surgery and Sports Medicine, Steamboat Orthopaedic Associates, P.C., Steamboat Springs, Colorado

AUTHORS

ELIZABETH ARENDT, MD
Professor, Department of Orthopaedic Surgery, University of Minnesota, Minneapolis, Minnesota

MATT BOLLIER, MD
Assistant Clinical Professor, Department of Orthopaedics and Rehabilitation, University of Iowa Hospitals and Clinics, Iowa City, Iowa

ROBERT BURKS, MD
Professor, Department of Orthopaedics, University of Utah, Salt Lake City, Utah

DAVIETTA BUTTY, BS
Department of Orthopedic Surgery, Rush University Medical Center, Chicago, Illinois

BRIAN J. COLE, MD, MBA
Professor, Department of Orthopedics; Department of Anatomy and Cell Biology; Section Head, Cartilage Restoration Center at Rush, Rush University Medical Center, Chicago, Illinois

TYLER R. CRAM, MA, ATC, OTC
Research Associate, The Steadman Clinic, Vail, Colorado

DIANE DAHM, MD
Associate Professor, Department of Orthopaedic Surgery, Mayo Clinic, Rochester, Minnesota

JAKE DAYNES, DO
Orthopaedic Sports Medicine Fellow, OrthoIndy, Greenwood, Indiana

KYLE DUCHMAN, MD
Department of Orthopaedics and Rehabilitation, University of Iowa Hospitals and Clinics, Iowa City, Iowa

JACK FARR, MD
Director, Department of Orthopedic Surgery, Cartilage Restoration Center of Indiana, Greenwood, Indiana

LAURIE ANNE HIEMSTRA, MD, PhD, FRCSC
Banff Sport Medicine, Banff, Alberta, Canada; Department of Surgery, University of Calgary, Calgary, Alberta, Canada

MELODY HRUBES, MD
Department of Orthopaedic Surgery, UIC Sports Medicine Center, Chicago, Illinois

MARK R. HUTCHINSON, MD
Professor of Orthopaedics and Sports Medicine, Department of Orthopedic Surgery, University of Illinois at Chicago, Chicago, Illinois

CHRISTOPHER IRVING, MD
Banff Sport Medicine, Banff, Alberta, Canada

EVAN W. JAMES, BS
Research Assistant, Center for Outcomes-based Orthopaedic Research, Steadman Philippon Research Institute, Vail, Colorado

SARAH KERSLAKE, BPhty (Hons)
Banff Sport Medicine, Banff, Alberta, Canada; Department of Physical Therapy, University of Alberta, Edmonton, Alberta, Canada

JASON L. KOH, MD
Chairman, Department of Orthopaedic Surgery; Board of Directors Endowed Chair, NorthShore University HealthSystem; Clinical Associate Professor, University of Chicago Pritzker School of Medicine, Chicago, Illinois

RAJ KULLAR, MD
Fellow and Visiting Instructor, Department of Orthopaedics, University of Utah, Salt Lake City, Utah

ROBERT F. LAPRADE, MD, PhD
Chief Medical Officer, The Steadman Clinic; Steadman Philippon Research Institute, Vail, Colorado

JONATHAN D. LESTER, MD
Resident, Department of Orthopaedic Surgery, University of Illinois at Chicago, Chicago, Illinois

TERRY L. NICOLA, MD, MS
Department of Orthopaedic Surgery, UIC Sports Medicine Center, Chicago, Illinois

CLAYTON W. NUELLE, MD
Department of Orthopaedic Surgery, University of Missouri, Columbia, Missouri

ANDREAS C. PLACKIS, BS
Department of Orthopaedic Surgery, University of Missouri, Columbia, Missouri

MATTHEW T. RASMUSSEN, BS
Research Assistant, Department of BioMedical Engineering, Steadman Philippon Research Institute, Vail, Colorado

JEFFREY REAGAN, MD
Fellow and Visiting Instructor, Department of Orthopaedics, University of Utah, Salt Lake City, Utah

DAVID RUPIPER, MD
Clinical Associate of Radiology, Department of Radiology, University of Chicago, Chicago, Illinois

BRYAN M. SALTZMAN, MD
Resident, Department of Orthopedic Surgery, Rush University Medical Center, Chicago, Illinois

SETH L. SHERMAN, MD
Department of Orthopaedic Surgery, University of Missouri, Columbia, Missouri

G. SCOTT STACY, MD
Associate Professor of Radiology; Chief, Section of Musculoskeletal Imaging, Department of Radiology, University of Chicago, Chicago, Illinois

CORY STEWART, MD
Department of Orthopaedic Surgery and Rehabilitation Medicine, University of Chicago Medicine & Biological Sciences, Chicago, Illinois

STEPHEN THOMAS, MD
Assistant Professor of Radiology, Department of Radiology, University of Chicago, Chicago, Illinois

JONATHAN N. WATSON, MD
Resident, Department of Orthopaedic Surgery, University of Illinois at Chicago, Chicago, Illinois

THOMAS WUERZ, MD
Sports Medicine Fellow, Department of Orthopedic Surgery, Rush University Medical Center, Chicago, Illinois

ADAM B. YANKE, MD
Sports Medicine Fellow, Department of Orthopedic Surgery, Rush University Medical Center, Chicago, Illinois

Contents

physical examination, and achieving an appropriate diagnosis and treatment approach. This clinical review provides an assessment framework and a guide for neuromuscular function testing, and an overview of the causes and treatments of AKP in this challenging patient population.

Patellar instability is a common injury that can result in significant limitations of activity and long-term arthritis. There is a high risk of recurrence in patients and operative management is often indicated. Advances in the understanding of patellofemoral anatomy, such as knowledge about the medial patellofemoral ligament, tibial tubercle-trochlear groove distance, and trochlear dysplasia may allow improved surgical management of patellar instability. However, techniques such as MPFL reconstruction are technically demanding and may result in significant complication. The role of trochleoplasty remains unclear.

The approach to treating cartilage defects of the patellofemoral joint hinges on appropriate clinical indications. Multiple surgical treatments can achieve promising clinical results. Factors that affect the outcome of patellofemoral chondral lesions include characteristics specific to the defect as well as general overall patient features. Outcomes of patellofemoral chondral defects have been promising and continue to improve. This article focuses on methods that have worked well in the authors' practice and that are also widely used. The goal is to create an algorithm that aids clinicians in treating this patient population.

 Video of an MPFL reconstruction with semitendinosis autograft accompanies this article

Patellar instability is a common problem, and medial patellofemoral ligament (MPFL) injury is inherent with traumatic patellar dislocations. Initial nonoperative management is focused on reconditioning and strengthening the dynamic stabilizers of the patella. For those patients who progress to recurrent instability, further investigation into the predisposing factors is required. MPFL reconstruction is indicated in patients with recurrent instability and insufficient medial restraint due to MPFL injury. A technique of MPFL reconstruction is outlined. This procedure may also be performed in combination with other realignment procedures.

Distal realignment can be used with or without proximal stabilization in cases of patellofemoral instability, cartilage lesions of the lateral and distal patellofemoral joint, or cases of lateral patellofemoral overload or tilt. Ante-romedialization of the tibial tubercle allows for multiplanar adjustments while providing a long, flat osteotomy that optimizes bone healing and screw placement. In cases of patella alta, distalization can be incorporated during the osteotomy.

CLINICS IN SPORTS MEDICINE

RELATED INTEREST

Orthopedic Clinics of North America, April 2014 (Vol. 45, No. 2)
Foot and Ankle Clinics of North America, September 2013 (Vol. 18, No. 3)

DOWNLOAD Free App!

Review Articles
THE CLINICS

NOW AVAILABLE FOR YOUR iPhone and iPad

Foreword

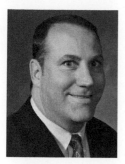

Mark D. Miller, MD
Consulting Editor

Dr. Meininger has done an excellent job in assembling an outstanding group of expert knee surgeons to cover the entire gambit of patellofemoral problems and solutions. He has put together a logical sequence of articles that, as the title suggests, will help us to understand the patellofemoral joint and patellofemoral surgery. After several introductory articles on anatomy, examination, and imaging, one chapter addresses the dreaded topic of anterior knee pain. This is followed by several chapters on treatment of patellofemoral instability–to include proximal, distal, and trochlear based procedures. Chondral injuries and DJD are also addressed and the treatise concludes with a thorough review of patellofemoral rehabilitation, which is often the mainstay for treating patellofemoral problems.

In sum, this issue should indeed help us better understand the Patellofemoral joint– perhaps a better understanding will allow us to better educate ourselves and our patients with these sometimes challenging problems. Thank you Dr. Meininger!

Mark D. Miller, MD
Division of Sports Medicine
Department of Orthopaedic Surgery
University of Virginia

James Madison University
Miller Review Course
400 Ray C. Hunt Drive, Suite 330
Charlottesville, VA 22908-0159, USA

E-mail address:
MDM3P@hscmail.mcc.virginia.edu

Preface

Understanding the Patellofemoral Joint: From Instability to Arthroplasty

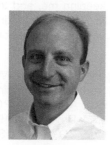

Alexander K. Meininger, MD
Editor

It is both an honor and a pleasure to be invited to serve as an editor for *Clinics in Sports Medicine*. For me, disorders of the patellofemoral joint are a distinct passion and clinical interest; one that is ever expanding with knowledge and expertise. I will never forget my colleague-in-training's statement, "I don't want to get involved in that crazy patient's kneecaps," as representative of what often appears as a clinical enigma. Much has been gained in the understanding of the patellofemoral joint thanks to organizations such as the Patellofemoral Study Group and the Arthroscopy Association of North America. I am grateful to assemble many of those same leaders in this issue.

Part one begins with Dr Seth Sherman's insightful review of the anatomy and biomechanics of a complex articulation. My mentor and astute clinician, Dr Mark Hutchinson, follows with his summation of the signs and symptoms of patellofemoral disorders to be found in the physical examination. The team of musculoskeletal radiologists assembled by Dr Scott Stacy is second to none and their task to summarize the radiology of the patellofemoral joint was daunting to say the least.

Dr Laurie Hiemstra brings an insightful review of anterior knee pain to what many consider a frustrating constellation of symptoms. A recognized leader in the field of cartilage restoration, Dr Brian Cole relays his state-of-the-art approach to the patellar chondral injury. Another mentor and the greatest contributor to my passion for patellofemoral disease, Dr Jason Koh, generously shares his insights on patellofemoral instability.

A renowned team, including Dr Robert Burks, Dr Matt Bolier, Dr Robert LaPrade, and Dr Jack Farr, summarize indications and pearls for successful outcomes when employing challenging patellofemoral techniques. Last, Dr Terry Nicola elegantly summarizes rehabilitation of the patellofemoral joint, equally as important as technique.

Clin Sports Med 33 (2014) xiii–xiv
http://dx.doi.org/10.1016/j.csm.2014.05.001   sportsmed.theclinics.com
0278-5919/14/$ – see front matter © 2014 Elsevier Inc. All rights reserved.

"Understanding the Patellofemoral Joint" seeks to do just that: elucidate for clinicians, surgeons, and sports medicine specialists the anatomy, biomechanics, pathophysiology, and treatment algorithms for disorders affecting the patellofemoral joint space.

This issue wouldn't have been accomplished without the contributions of each author. The time and dedication of clinicians to produce thoughtful articles are what make the *Clinics in Sports Medicine* such a success. Thanks to our Editor, Dr Mark Miller, for allowing me this opportunity to serve. Similarly, a special thank-you is due to Jennifer Flynn-Briggs and Donald Mumford at Elsevier for keeping me, and the issue, on task and on time. Last, I give thanks to my beautiful wife, Angie, for granting me the time and understanding to fulfill my academic pursuits. Without her support, none of these accomplishments could be realized.

Alexander K. Meininger, MD
Orthopaedic Surgery and Sports Medicine
Steamboat Orthopaedic Associates, P.C.
940 Central Park Drive, Suite 190
Steamboat Springs, CO 80487, USA

E-mail address:
DrAlex@steamboatortho.com

Patellofemoral Anatomy and Biomechanics

Seth L. Sherman, MD*, Andreas C. Plackis, BS, Clayton W. Nuelle, MD

KEYWORDS

- Patella anatomy • Trochlea anatomy • Patella pathology • Trochlea pathology
- Patellofemoral anatomy • Patellofemoral biomechanics

KEY POINTS

- Patellofemoral disorders encompass a large spectrum of disease including patellofemoral pain, instability, focal chondral disease, and arthritis.
- Most patellofemoral disorders are the result of aberrant anatomy (ie, soft tissue injury, bony malalignment) that predisposes the patient to biomechanical abnormalities (ie, patella maltracking).
- There are multiple bony and soft tissue stabilizers to the patella. Soft tissue stabilizers (ie, medial patellofemoral ligament [MPFL]) are critical from 0° to 20° of knee flexion, while the trochlear groove provides stability at greater than 20°.
- Abnormalities of dynamic muscle strength (ie, vastus medialis obliquus [VMO]), static soft tissue restraint (ie, MPFL, lateral retinaculum), patella height and tilt, trochlear morphology, and tibial tubercle position have profound effects on patellofemoral kinematics and may lead to clinical dysfunction.

INTRODUCTION

A thorough understanding of the basic anatomy and biomechanics of the patellofemoral joint is critical for any clinician who wishes to treat the broad spectrum of disorders that can occur.

EPIDEMIOLOGY

In orthopedic and musculoskeletal clinics, evaluation of patellofemoral pain encompasses up to 10% of all visits and has been reported as high as 30% in the 13- to 19 year-old age group.[1,2] Patellofemoral disorders comprise nearly 25% of all knee injuries.[3–5] They are more common in women than in men.[6] The incidence of primary

Disclosures: No external funds were used in the completion of this text, and none of the authors received payments or services from a third party for any aspect of this work.
Department of Orthopaedic Surgery, University of Missouri, 1100 Virginia Avenue, DC953.00, Columbia, MO 65212, USA
* Corresponding author.
E-mail address: dr.seth.sherman@gmail.com

patellar dislocation is 5.8 cases per 100,000 population, and up to 29 cases per 100,000 population in patients aged 10 to 17 years.[7] Chondral lesions have been reported in upwards of 60% of patients who underwent routine knee arthroscopies.[8] Patellofemoral pathology has a significant impact on time lost from sport or work.[9]

SPECTRUM OF DISEASE

Patellofemoral disorders encompass a large spectrum of disease, including patellofemoral pain, instability, focal chondral disease, and arthritis. Dysfunction can be the direct result of trauma (ie, patella dislocation) or insidious in nature (ie, patellofemoral pain, arthritis). Most patellofemoral disorders are the result of aberrant anatomy (ie, bony malalignment) that predisposes the patient to biomechanical abnormalities (ie, patella maltracking). Successful treatment requires an understanding of the anatomy/biomechanics of the joint, in order to recognize and correct common patterns that lead to patellofemoral dysfunction. Anatomic and biomechanic abnormalities may be addressed nonoperatively (ie, dynamic strengthening/stability, bracing) or operatively (ie, tubercle osteotomy, MPFL repair/reconstruction, patellofemoral cartilage restoration or resurfacing, or trochleoplasty). A comprehensive treatment plan must address both the biology and the biomechanics for optimal results.

ANATOMY
Osseous Anatomy of the Patella

The patella is the largest sesamoid bone in the body. It resides within the trochlear groove of the distal femur and links the extensor mechanism through connections to the quadriceps tendon at its superior pole and the patellar tendon at its inferior pole.

The patella is convex on its anterior surface, but is divided by a longitudinal median ridge on the articular side. The patella has 7 total facets, but is primarily divided into the 2 large medial and lateral facets.

The lateral facet is typically longer and more sloped to match the lateral femoral condyle, while the medial facet is smaller, with a shorter but consequently steeper slope.[10] The Wiberg classification delineates 4 different types based on the location of the median ridge (**Fig. 1**).[11] The primary blood supply to the patella occurs from a complex arterial plexus that forms an anastomotic ring surrounding the patella.[12,13] Patellar articular cartilage is the thickest found in the body, measuring up to 7 mm.[14]

Patella cartilage has much greater congruency in the axial plane compared with the sagittal plane, contributing to the gliding capability of the joint itself. Contour of the cartilage does not always follow that of its underlying subchondral bone.[15]

The articular surface is only present on the superior two-thirds of the patella, as the distal pole serves as the patellar tendon insertion and is extra-articular (**Fig. 2**).

Osseous Anatomy of the Trochlea

The trochlea is formed by the anterior aspect of the distal femur. It has a centralized trochlear groove (TG) with associated medial and lateral facets.

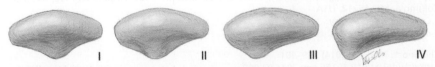

Fig. 1. Illustration demonstrating the Wiberg classification of patella anatomy.

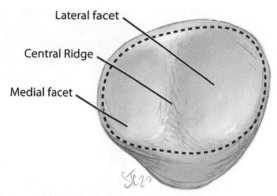

Fig. 2. Illustration demonstrating the posterior aspect of the patella, which consists of carti-lage over the proximal two-thirds and an extra-articular portion along the distal one-third of the patella.

The lateral facet is larger and extends more proximally than the medial facet. The depth of a normal TG is 5.2 mm, with the lateral femoral condyle being 3.4 mm higher than the medial femoral condyle in the axial plane.[10]

The TG deepens as it extends distally and deviates lateral before it terminates at the femoral notch. The facets transition into the medial and lateral femoral condyles.[16]

The depth of the TG can be measured by the sulcus angle (**Fig. 3**).

Trochlear dysplasia is characterized by a loss of the normal concave anatomy and depth of the TG, creating a flat trochlea with highly asymmetrical facets. This frequently predisposes to patellar dislocation during knee flexion secondary to the loss of restraint of the patella within the groove.

Dejour and colleagues[17] quantified trochlear dysplasia radiographically and defined the trochlear bump, deemed pathologic when greater than 3 mm, and the trochlear depth, deemed pathologic at 4 mm or less (**Figs. 4** and **5**). The lateral condyle forms

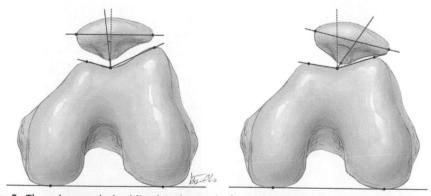

Fig. 3. The sulcus angle (*red lines*) is the angle formed in the axial plane from the highest point on the lateral facet, to the trochlear groove, to the highest point on the medial facet. An angle of 138° represents normal anatomy, with an angle of 150° or greater representing an abnormally shallow groove. The congruence angle (*green lines*) is formed from a line drawn through the apex of the trochlear groove with a line through the lowest point on the articular ridge of the patella. A value of -6° represents normal anatomy, while a value greater than 16° represents an abnormal patellofemoral articulation. Patellar tilt (*blue lines*) is the angle formed by a line drawn parallel to the posterior femoral condyles and a line drawn through the transverse axis of the patella.

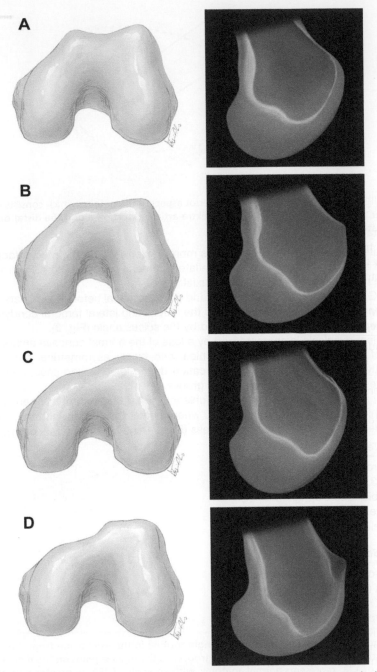

Fig. 4. Illustration depicting the Dejour classification of trochlear dysplasia with the corresponding lateral radiograph of each type.

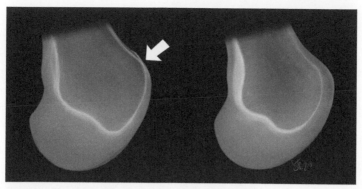

Fig. 5. Illustration depicting the crossover sign (*white arrow*), as seen on a lateral radiograph in the setting of trochlear dysplasia.

the lateral wall of the patellofemoral articulation and is the primary restraint to lateral patellar translation once the patella is deeply engaged in the groove.[18] Hypoplasia of either the medial or lateral femoral condyle can also contribute to abnormal trochlear anatomy and subsequent patellofemoral articulation abnormality.

ANATOMY OF PATELLOFEMORAL SOFT TISSUE STRUCTURES
Quadriceps Mechanism

The quadriceps mechanism is an important contributor to dynamic patellofemoral joint stability. It is formed by the convergence of 4 muscles: the rectus femoris, vastus medialis, vastus lateralis, and vastus intermedius.

The tendon results as a confluence of these individual muscle tendons 5 cm to 8 cm superior to the patella and subsequently inserts on the proximal pole of the patella. The femoral nerves supply the muscles of the quadriceps mechanism.

Patella Tendon

Arising from the inferior pole of the patella, the patellar tendon has an average length of 4.6 cm (3.5 cm–5.5 cm), and width between 24 mm and 33 mm.[19] Its insertion is found on the tibial tubercle, slightly lateralized in relation to the long axis of the tibia. Separating the posterior part of the patellar tendon from the synovial membrane of the joint is the infrapatellar fat pad, whereas a bursa separates the tendon from the tibia more distally.

Medial Soft Tissues

Medial soft tissues include the vastus medialis obliquus (VMO), medial patellofemoral ligament (MPFL), the medial patellotibial ligament, and the medial retinaculum (**Fig. 6**). The VMO is one of the most important muscles contributing to patellar mechanics, as it is the primary dynamic restraint to lateral tracking of the patella.[14] In a cadaveric study, VMO weakness was found to increase lateral patellar translation when simulated from 0° to 15° of flexion.[20]

VMO hypoplasia or dysplasia is a major cause of dynamic patella instability. VMO strengthening is a mainstay of rehabilitation for many patellofemoral disorders.

The MPFL is the primary passive restraint to lateral patellofemoral translation. The MPFL contributes up to 60% of the restraint to lateral patellar displacement at 0° to 30° of flexion and is vital to the maintenance of patellar stability.[21–23] MPFL laxity may be the result of congenital abnormalities, or due to traumatic lateral subluxation or dislocation events of the patella.

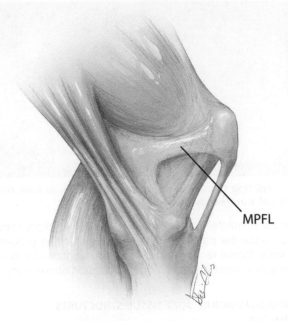

MPFL

Fig. 6. Illustration of the soft tissue restraints to the patella on the medial aspect of the knee, including the medial patellofemoral ligament.

The MPFL originates at a point just proximal and posterior to the medial epicondyle and distal to the adductor tubercle. It inserts on the proximal and medial surface of the patella.[21] The mean length of the MPFL is 53 mm to 55 mm, whereas its width may range from 3 mm to 30 mm and widen at its attachments.[19,21]

Lateral Soft Tissues

The lateral soft tissue restraint to the patella is comprised of multiple layers but is frequently divided into a superficial and deep layer. The superficial layer is composed of the oblique lateral retinaculum, while the deep layer is composed of oblique and transverse fibers, specifically the patellotibial band and the epicondylopatellar bands (**Fig. 7**).[24]

The lateral retinaculum is an important secondary stabilizer of lateral translation of the patella. In the setting of patella instability due to loss of medial soft tissue restraints, isolated surgical lateral release may worsen lateral patella instability, and/or cause iatrogenic medial patella instability.

Lateral retinacular tightness is a common cause of patellofemoral pain. This may result in lateral patella tilt, abnormally high forces between the lateral facet of the patella and the lateral trochlea, and degenerative changes over time.

Clinically, patellar tilt can be evaluated with the patient supine, the knee in full extension, and the quadriceps muscle relaxed. In a normal knee, there is no tenderness to palpation along the lateral patella facet, and the lateral edge of the patella can be gently lifted away from the lateral femoral condyle.

Patellar tilt may be measured radiographically by use of radiograph, computed tomography (CT), or magnetic resonance imaging (MRI). It can be on measured on an axial image by the angle formed by the posterior femoral condyles and the transverse patellar axis (see **Fig. 3**).[25] Normal patellar tilt is 2°, whereas abnormal patellar tilt is defined as greater than 5°.[14]

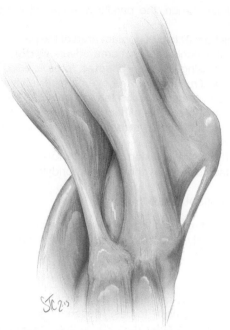

Fig. 7. Illustration depicting the soft tissue restraints to the patella on the lateral aspect of the knee.

Surgical lateral release may be indicated in the setting of isolated lateral patellofemoral pain and/or chondrosis from fixed patella tilt and lateral retinacular tightness that is refractory to conservative treatment.

BIOMECHANICS

Patellofemoral motion requires a complex interplay of the previously described bony and soft tissue structures. Anatomic abnormalities of the bones cause malalignment and may predispose patella maltracking. Abnormalities of the dynamic and static soft tissue structures have significant effects on patellofemoral biomechanics.

As a sesamoid bone, the patella enhances the mechanical advantage of the extensor mechanism.

Functioning as a lever, the patella acts to magnify either force or displacement, depending on the activity, and helps to increase the moment arm of the quadriceps. This decreases the amount of quadriceps force necessary to extend the knee.[14]

Normal Patella Tracking

Different components of the patellofemoral joint play crucial stabilizing roles throughout the normal motion arc. From 0° to 30° of knee flexion, the primary restraints to lateral patellofemoral translation are the soft tissues mentioned previously, particularly the MPFL.[26]

In full knee extension, there are minimal posterior directed forces on the patella. The patella rests in a slightly lateralized position.

Due to the patella's unique articular surface orientation, a medial patellar shift is produced when the knee begins to flex. This centers the patella as it engages the trochlea groove.[14]

At 20° to 30° of knee flexion, the patella is engaged in the trochlea, providing increased stability.[27]

As flexion increases from 0° to 60°, contact area of the patella increases, and moves from distal to proximal. Trochlea contact area advances distally.[18]

There is also an increasing posterior directed force exerted from the patellar and quadriceps tendons, which increases the overall joint reactive force (**Fig. 8**). Once the knee flexes past 90°, the quadriceps tendon contacts the trochlea and absorbs some of the joint reaction force. This either causes the force to level off or decreases as the quadriceps tendon becomes responsible for some of the total joint reaction force and contact area.[14,28,29]

Between 90° and 135° of knee flexion, the patella rotates, and the ridge that divides the medial and odd facets engages the femoral condyle.[24]

MEASUREMENTS OF OSSEOUS RESTRAINT

The coronal, sagittal, and axial plane alignment of the patella can be measured clinically and radiographically. Aberrant anatomy predisposes to biomechanical abnormalities.

Coronal and Axial Planes

Clinically, the quadriceps or Q-angle plays a significant role in evaluation of patellofemoral tracking and patellofemoral forces. Measurement of the Q angle is demonstrated in **Fig. 9**. A Q angle greater than 20° is considered abnormal and may lead

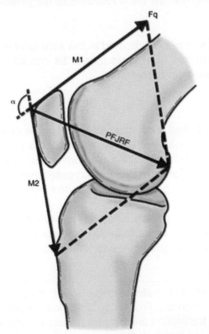

Fig. 8. Illustration depicting the patellofemoral joint reaction force (PFJRF). The PFJRF becomes higher as the knee flexion angle increases. In complete extension, M1 and M2 are in opposite directions, but in the same plane; the resultant PFJRF is almost zero. As flexion increases, M1 and M2 converge, and the vector PFJRF increases. (*From* DeJour D, Saggin PRF. Disorders of the patellofemoral joint. In: Scott WN. Insall & Scott surgery of the knee. Philadelphia: Elsevier/Churchill Livingstone, 2012; with permission.)

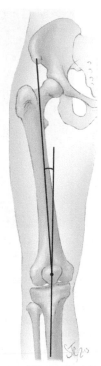

Fig. 9. Illustration depicting the measurement of the Q angle. The Q angle is measured by the intersection of a line drawn from the anterior superior iliac spine through the center of the patella and a line from the tibial tubercle through the center of the patella.

to both increased lateral displacement force and increased patellar contact pressures.[30]

The mean Q angle typically measures 14° in men and 17° in women, with the gender difference being the result of a wider pelvis in women, leading to an increase in knee valgus alignment.[31]

The tibial tuberosity–trochlear groove (TT-TG) distance is a more accurate method of quantifying axial anatomy of the patellofemoral articulation (**Fig. 10**). The mean TT-TG in normal patients ranges from 10 mm to 13 mm, with a value greater than 15 mm associated with increased risk of patellar instability.[32] The congruence angle is a static radiographic measure of patella position in the axial plane (see **Fig. 3**).

Sagittal Plane

Abnormal patellar height has been shown to contribute to patellar instability and subsequent recurrent patellar dislocation.[30,33] In addition, abnormalities in patellar height relative to the joint line may affect overall patellofemoral function and result in pain syndromes.[34,35]

A high-riding patella, or patella alta, results in more knee flexion prior to the patella engaging the trochlea, which may result in chondromalacia or an increased risk of dislocation episodes.[30,33] A low-riding patella, or patella baja, results in increased joint reactive forces on the patella, which may lead to motion limitation and early patellofemoral arthritis (**Fig. 11**).[35]

Numerous methods have been described to evaluate patellar height, including: the Insall-Salvati index,[36] The Blackburne-Peel index,[34] and the Caton-Deschamps index.[37]

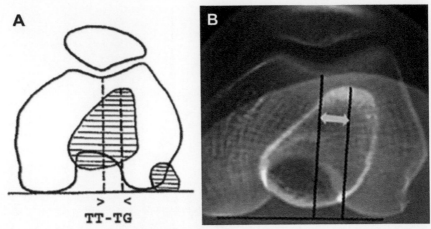

Fig. 10. (*A*) Illustration demonstrating how to calculate the tibial tuberosity–trochlear groove distance. (*B*) CT scan demonstrating how to calculate the TT-TG distance. The TT-TG is calculated by the superimposition of 2 axial CT or MRI slices: one through the apex of the trochlear groove and one through the center of the proximal tibial tuberosity. The distance between these 2 perpendicular lines is measured, as referenced from the posterior condylar line of the distal femur. (*From* Sherman SL, Erickson BJ, Cvetanovich GL, et al. Tibial tuberosity osteotomy: indications, techniques, and outcomes. Am J Sports Med. 2013 Nov 6. [Epub ahead of print]; with permission.)

The Caton-Deschamps index is a widely used method, as its value does not vary with knee flexion. Unlike Insall-Salvati, this measurement changes with tibial tubercle osteotomy (ie, distalization). This allows the surgeon to use the measurement to accurately template and implement the desired amount of correction of patella height during surgery. It is measured by dividing 2 lengths: (1) the distance between the distal most aspect of the articular surface of the patella and the superior anterior angle of the tibia, and (2) the length of the articular surface of the patella (**Fig. 12**).

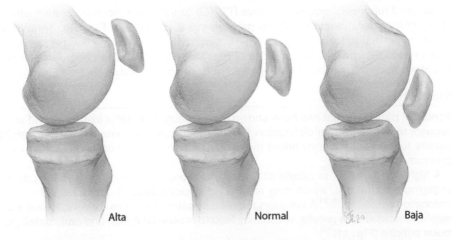

Fig. 11. Illustration of a lateral view of the knee depicting: patella alta, normal patella height, and patella baja.

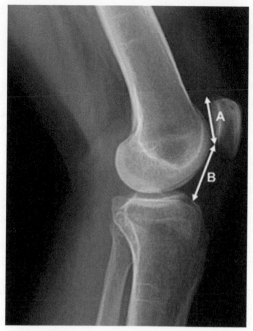

Fig. 12. Lateral radiograph exhibiting the Caton-Deschamps index (B/A): the ratio of the distance of the inferior aspect of the articular surface of the patella and the anterosuperior angle of the tibia's outline (B) and the length of the articular surface of the patella (A). (*From* Sherman SL, Erickson BJ, Cvetanovich GL, et al. Tibial tuberosity osteotomy: indications, techniques, and outcomes. Am J Sports Med. 2013 Nov 6. [Epub ahead of print]; with permission.)

Abnormal Patella Tracking

Central tracking within a normal TG and the absence of any patellar tilt are required for normal patellofemoral motion.[38]

Various previously described anatomic abnormalities can lead to altered patellofemoral forces and abnormal patella tracking. Clinically, these anatomic and biomechanical abnormalities may manifest as patellofemoral pain, instability, chondrosis, or a combination.

Critically important factors to consider include
Hypoplasia or weakness of the VMO
Injury or absence of static medial soft tissue restraints (MPFL)
Trochlear dysplasia
Abnormally high Q angle and increased TT-TG (or TT-posterior cruciate ligament [PCL])
Patella tilt with tight lateral retinaculum
Patella alta or baja

SUMMARY

Patellofemoral disorders are common. There is a broad spectrum of disease, ranging from patellofemoral pain and instability to focal cartilage disease and arthritis. Regardless of the specific condition, abnormal anatomy and biomechanics are often the root cause of patellofemoral dysfunction. A thorough understanding of normal patellofemoral anatomy and biomechanics is critical for the treating physician. Recognizing and addressing abnormal anatomy will optimize patellofemoral biomechanics and may ultimately translate into clinical success.

REFERENCES

1. Kannus P, Aho H, Järvinen M, et al. Computerized recording of visits to an outpatient sports clinic. Am J Sports Med 1987;15:79–85.
2. Blond L, Hansen L. Patellofemoral pain syndrome in athletes: a 5.7-year retrospective follow-up study of 250 athletes. Acta Orthop Belg 1998;64:393–400.
3. Baquie P, Brukner P. Injuries presenting to an Australian sports medicine centre: a 12-month study. Clin J Sport Med 1997;7:28–31.
4. Taunton JE, Ryan MB, Clement DB, et al. A retrospective case-control analysis of 2002 running injuries. Br J Sports Med 2002;36:95–101.
5. Lankhorst NE, Bierma-Zeinstra SM, van Middelkoop M. Factors associated with patellofemoral pain syndrome: a systematic review. Br J Sports Med 2013;47: 193–206.
6. Boling M, Padua D, Marshall S, et al. Gender differences in the incidence and prevalence of patellofemoral pain syndrome. Scand J Med Sci Sports 2010;20: 725–30.
7. Fithian DC, Paxton WE, Stone ML, et al. Epidemiology and natural history of acute patellar dislocation. Am J Sports Med 2004;32:1114–21.
8. Widuchowski W, Widuchowski J, Trzaska T. Articular cartilage defects: study of 25,124 knee arthroscoopies. Knee 2007;14(3):177–82.
9. Selfe J, Callaghan M, Ritchie E, et al. Targeted interventions for patellofemoral pain syndrome (TIPPS): classification of clinical subgroups. BMJ Open 2013; 3(9):e003795.
10. Walsh W. Recurrent dislocation of the knee in the adult. In: Delee J, Drez D, Miller M, editors. Delee and Drez's orthopaedic sports medicine. Philadelphia: Saunders; 2003. p. 1710–49.
11. Wiberg G. Roentgenographic and anatomic studies on the femoropatellar joint. Acta Orthop Scand 1941;12:319–410.
12. Scapinelli R. Blood supply of the human patella: its relation to ischaemic necrosis after fracture. J Bone Joint Surg Br 1967;49:563–70.
13. Bjorkstrom S, Goldie IF. A study of the arterial supply of the patella in the normal state, in chondromalacia patellae and in osteoarthrosis. Acta Orthop Scand 1980; 51:63–70.
14. Grelsamer RP, Proctor CS, Bazos AN. Evaluation of patellar shape in the sagittal plane. A clinical analysis. Am J Sports Med 1994;22:61.
15. Ahmed AM, Burke DL, Hyder A. Force analysis of the patellar mechanism. J Orthop Res 1987;5:6–85.
16. Merchant AC, Mercer RL, Jacobsen RH, et al. Roentgenographic analysis of patello-femoral congruence. J Bone Joint Surg Am 1974;56:1391.
17. Dejour H, Walch G, Nove-Josserand L, et al. Factors of patellar instability: an anatomic radiographic study. Knee Surg Sports Traumatol Arthrosc 1994;2:19–26.
18. White BJ, Sherman OH. Patellofemoral instability. Bull NYU Hosp Jt Dis 2009;67: 22–9.
19. Reider B, Marshall JL, Koslin B, et al. The anterior aspect of the knee joint. J Bone Joint Surg Am 1981;63:351–6.
20. Sakai N, Luo ZP, Rand JA, et al. The influence of weakness in the vastus medialis oblique muscle on the patellofemoral joint: an in vitro biomechanical study. Clin Biomech 2000;15:335–9.

21. Amis AA, Firer P, Mountney J, et al. Anatomy and biomechanics of the medial patellofemoral ligament. Knee 2003;10:215–20.
22. Conlan T, Garth WP Jr, Lemons JE. Evaluation of the medial soft-tissue restraints of the extensor mechanism of the knee. J Bone Joint Surg Am 1993;75:682–93.
23. Hautamaa PV, Fithian DC, Kaufman KR, et al. Medial soft tissue restraints in lateral patellar instability and repair. Clin Orthop Relat Res 1998;349:174–82.
24. Dejour D, Saggin P. Disorders of the patellofemoral joint. In: Scott N, editor. Insall & Scott surgery of the knee. Philadelphia: Elsevier; 2012. Chapter 61.
25. Canale S, Beaty J. Campbell's operative orthopaedics. St Louis (MO): Mosby; 2012.
26. Desio SM, Burks RT, Bachus KN. Soft tissue restraints to lateral patellar translation in the human knee. Am J Sports Med 1998;26:59–65.
27. Schepsis AA. Patellar instability [video]. In: Grana WA, editor. Orthopaedic Knowledge Online. 2007. Available at: http://www5.aaos.org/oko/description.cfm?topic=SPO004&referringPage=http://www5.aaos.org/oko/menus/topicAuthors.cfm.
28. Hungerford DS, Barry M. Biomechanics of the patellofemoral joint. Clin Orthop Relat Res 1979;144:9–15.
29. Cistac C, Cartier P. Diagnostic et traitment des desequilibres rotuliens du sportif. J Traumatol Sport 1986;3:92–7.
30. Aglietti P, Insall JN, Cerulli G. Patellar pain and incongruence. I: measurements of incongruence. Clin Orthop Relat Res 1983;176:217–24.
31. Phillips BB. Recurrent dislocations. In: Canale ST, editor. Campbell's operative orthopaedics. St Louis (MO): Mosby; 2003. p. 2377–449.
32. Balcarek P, Jung K, Frosch KH, et al. Value of the tibial tuberosity-trochlear groove distance in patellar instability in the young athlete. Am J Sports Med 2011;39(8):1756–61.
33. Simmons E Jr, Cameron JC. Patella alta and recurrent dislocation of the patella. Clin Orthop Relat Res 1992;274:265–9.
34. Blackburne JS, Peel TE. A new method of measuring patellar height. J Bone Joint Surg Br 1977;59:241–2.
35. Lancourt JE, Cristini JA. Patella alta and patella infera. Their etiological role in patellar dislocation, chondromalacia, and apophysitis of the tibial tubercle. J Bone Joint Surg Am 1975;57:1112–5.
36. Insall J, Salvati E. Patella position in the normal knee joint. Radiology 1971;101:101–4.
37. Caton J, Deschamps G, Chambat P, et al. Patella infera. Apropos of 128 cases. Rev Chir Orthop Reparatrice Appar Mot 1982;68:317–25.
38. Ramappa AJ, Apreleva M, Harrold FR, et al. The effects of medialization and anteromedialization of the tibial tubercle on patellofemoral mechanics and kinematics. Am J Sports Med 2006;34:749–56.

Physical Examination of the Patellofemoral Joint

 CrossMark

Jonathan D. Lester, MD*, Jonathan N. Watson, MD, Mark R. Hutchinson, MD

KEYWORDS

- Patellofemoral • Physical exam • PTFS • Q angle • Grind test • Glide test

KEY POINTS

- Examination of the patellofemoral joint can prove to be challenging.
- Although certain acute injuries such as patella fracture or tendon rupture can be diagnosed quickly, more chronic injuries such as patellar subluxation and patellofemoral pain syndrome are more difficult to diagnose because of the subtlety of the examination findings.
- The source of the problem can also vary, and must be identified to direct treatment.
- Adding to the complexity is that other structures around the knee may present with anterior knee pain and can be mistaken for patellofemoral abnormality, which is why the patellofemoral examination should be performed in the context of a complete knee examination.
- Performing a thorough and systematic examination of the patellofemoral joint can lead to optimal patient outcomes.

INTRODUCTION

Although the patellofemoral joint may seem simple at a glance, there is a wide range of abnormalities and potentially causative or contributive factors involved. A comprehensive examination can be challenging, given that these factors can be intrinsic to the patellofemoral joint itself or extrinsically related to other parts of the body. Contributing factors can be static or dynamic in nature, and may also be position dependent. Adding to the complexity of the patellofemoral examination is that many of the physical examination findings may be subtle, and may not always completely or directly correlate with symptoms. Experience is helpful; making a thorough examination of the patellofemoral joint a routine part of a good knee examination will give the clinician a good

Disclosures: None.
Department of Orthopaedic Surgery, University of Illinois at Chicago, 835 South Wolcott Avenue, Suite E-270, Chicago, IL 60612, USA
* Corresponding author.
E-mail address: jlester328@gmail.com

Clin Sports Med 33 (2014) 403–412
http://dx.doi.org/10.1016/j.csm.2014.03.002
0278-5919/14/$ – see front matter © 2014 Elsevier Inc. All rights reserved.

foundation for what is normal and what is not. Ultimately it is of great importance that the approach be systematic, complete, and detailed, to allow the clinician to identify all contributing factors, which in turn will lead to focused treatment and better outcomes for patients.

As is the case with much of orthopedics, examination of the patellofemoral joint is most useful when performed in association with a good history. The value of the physical examination is directly linked to its correlation with symptomatology. Knowledge about the symptoms' onset, location, character, and any aggravating or alleviating factors will help with diagnosis. Before assuming a mechanical patellofemoral diagnosis, a good clinician will assure that the patient does not have fevers, chills, redness, or swelling that might represent infection. The patient should be asked about other joint involvement that might represent systemic or rheumatologic disease. Night pain is a classic red-flag symptom that should alert the clinician to the possible diagnosis of tumor. If there is a low suspicion regarding these other issues, the clinician can focus on the more classic musculoskeletal diagnoses.

Anterior knee pain is a common but nonspecific complaint that may be associated with cartilage damage, tendinopathy, bone injury, or instability. The classic presentation of chondromalacia patella includes anterior knee complaints that worsen with sitting for an extended period of time, such as sitting in a theater, riding on an airplane, or taking an extended car trip. Chondromalacia or patellofemoral arthrosis is also classically exacerbated with deep squats and climbing stairs. Pain along the extensor mechanism exacerbated by explosive starts or jumping should alert the examiner to the potential of tendinopathy. Patients with patellofemoral instability will often complain of a giving-way sensation in their knee or that their knee feels like it is about to go out of place, or may provide a history of a dislocation event. Ultimately a careful assessment of the history provided by the patient will usually narrow the potential differential diagnosis and allow the examiner to be particularly thorough in that portion of the physical examination.

A comprehensive examination should be performed on each patient, thus enabling the examiner to gain more experience in detecting the subtle findings often associated with the patellofemoral joint. The examination should include an assessment of gait and overall lower extremity alignment. Every lower extremity examination should include an evaluation of the lumbar spine and neurologic system for the potential of radiculopathy and referred pain. No knee examination should be considered complete in the absence of an assessment of the hip and core function; this is especially true for the pediatric patient who may have hip abnormality such as slipped capital femoral epiphysis or Legg-Calves-Perthes disease referring pain to the knee. It is equally important for the female patient for whom alignment, core strength, and motor function can play key roles in both the causation and treatment of patellofemoral problems.

OVERVIEW

Although the sequence of examination maneuvers may be altered based on the individual, generally it should be performed in a systematic manner so as not to overlook any maneuvers. The authors believe that the most efficient manner of examining the patellofemoral joint is by dividing the examination into patient positions: (1) standing, (2) sitting, and (3) lying. The examination in each position should begin with inspection both statically and dynamically, followed by palpation, finishing with specific maneuvers. These specific maneuvers can sequentially test the most common diagnoses leading to patellofemoral complaints.

STANDING

The standing portion of the patellofemoral examination consists of static observation in addition to dynamic observation during squats and gait. It is important that the subject changes into shorts that do not cover the knees and removes both socks and shoes to aid in the examination. The latter is key to making an assessment of foot alignment (particularly looking for pes planus), which has been directly related to knee pain in some patients.

After a general inspection for bruising, redness, swelling, and posttraumatic or postsurgical scars, the physician should observe overall limb alignment with the feet together. Does the patient have a significant varus alignment (bow-legged) or valgus alignment (knock-kneed)? Traditionally, alignment at the knee is quantified by the Q-angle, which is the angle formed between a line from the anterosuperior iliac spine (ASIS) to the patella and another from the patella to the middle of the anterior tibial tuberosity (**Fig. 1**). A larger Q-angle represents a larger laterally directed force on the patella. Theoretically this could increase the risk of patellar subluxation and dislocation or lead to patella maltracking, which may be implicated in patellofemoral pain syndrome (PTFS). An increase in Q-angle can be a result of malalignment at any point in the lower extremity. It is important to not only observe genu valgum in the knee but also increased femoral anteversion, suggested by inward pointing or "winking" patellae, tibial external rotation, and hind-foot valgus. Some studies have reported a Q-angle greater than 16° as being a risk factor for developing PTFS.[1,2] However, others have failed to find a correlation between Q-angle and either PTFS or patellar

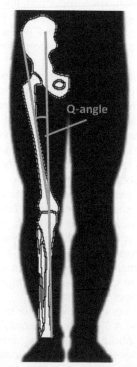

Fig. 1. The Q-angle is defined as the angle formed between a line from the anterosuperior iliac spine to the patella and another from the patella to the middle of the anterior tibial tuberosity.

subluxation.[3] The discrepancy between the studies likely is due to the poor interobserver reliability of measuring the Q-angle. If the patella is subluxated, the measurement will be too low. If the patient's lower extremity is internally rotated at the hip, the measurement will be too high. Some investigators have tried to minimize this effect by assessing the Q-angle with the knee in a flexed position. However, more important than the specific Q-angle measurement is the basic knowledge that alignment plays a direct role in the function of the patellofemoral joint.

In addition to alignment, any leg-length discrepancy can be seen in the static standing position. The examiner should inspect the patient from posterior to assess the height of the iliac crests. Direct measurements of leg lengths can be performed by measuring from the ASIS to the medial malleolus of the ankle. During this static upright inspection of the knee, it is also important to make note of the relative height of the patella. Patella alta has been associated with instability, and patella baja has been associated with chondromalacia patella. Inspection of the standing patient from the side may demonstrate inability to fully extend at the knee, which has been correlated with patellofemoral arthrosis, or knee hyperextension (recurvatum), which may represent generalized ligamentous laxity and an increased risk of patella instability.

After completing the static assessment, the patellofemoral joint must be observed dynamically. This evaluation is usually accomplished with both single and double leg squats in addition to observation of gait. Malalignment during squats can indicate weakness in the gluteus (core) or quadriceps (particularly vastus medialis obliquus) muscles, and may be exacerbated by poor motor control in the ankle. Previous studies have shown that patients with poor dynamic muscle control tend to have pelvic drop, hip adduction, hip internal rotation, knee abduction, tibial external rotation, and ankle hyperpronation, which in turn has been associated with PTFS.[4–6] Although quadriceps weakness has traditionally been associated with PTFS, weakness of the hip abductors and external rotators may play an even more important role.[7] Hamstring tightness has also been implicated.[8–10]

While observing the patella itself, close attention should be paid to actual patellar tracking, looking specifically for the presence of a J-sign. This finding exemplifies that when the knee is flexed, the patella is forced centrally to track in the trochlea of the femur. As the knee approaches full extension, the centralizing forces have less of a mechanical advantage, and a patella that is prone to track laterally will jump out of the groove and move laterally nearer full extension.[11] Palpation of the patella during dynamic squatting may reveal crepitus and grinding, indicating the underlying patellofemoral arthrosis or chondromalacia.

The final phase of dynamic patellofemoral assessment in the upright patient is a brief gait analysis. The patient should be inspected from both anterior and posterior views while walking forward, backward, on the heels, and on the toes along a stable flat surface. The latter 2 portions of the gait analysis are a simple assessment of general lower extremity function. Assessment of gait while walking backward is an effective way to assess patient compliance, because it is difficult to fake a limp walking backwards. The most important part of the gait analysis is inspecting the gait while looking from the front and back of the patient.

An antalgic gait or limp may represent pain, motor dysfunction, leg-length discrepancy, or core motor weakness. A Trendelenburg gait, or a drop in the contralateral pelvis, may be seen with hip abductor weakness. Some patients may walk with a quadriceps avoidance gait whereby the patient avoids knee extension, which can be related to any abnormality along the extensor mechanism. Positive findings during gait analysis should be more specifically targeted during the seated or supine portions of the examination.

As noted previously, it is important for the clinician to consider systemic issues such as infection, rheumatologic problems, or tumors as potential causes of anterior knee pain. In addition to these factors generally screened through history, another important factor that should be considered in all patients with patellofemoral problems is the potential contribution of generalized ligamentous laxity, which has been associated with PTFS.[9,12,13] The patient can be screened for a history of other joint dislocations or the feeling that they are "double jointed." Examination findings (Beighton criteria) consistent with generalized ligamentous laxity include the ability to rest the palms of the hands flat on the floor with forward flexion of the trunk and the knees fully extended, passive dorsiflexion of the small fingers beyond 90°, passive apposition of the thumbs to the volar aspects of the forearm, hyperextension of the elbows beyond 10°, and hyperextension of the knee beyond 10° (**Box 1**).

SITTING

The patient is then examined in a seated position with the knees flexed over the examining table. The knee should again be observed for any abnormalities. Any skin changes and any significant swelling in comparison with the asymptomatic limb should be noted. Differences in quadriceps muscle bulk, the vastus medialis (VMO) in particular, can often be seen at this point. The VMO has been shown to play an important role in patellar stabilization.[14,15] The examiner can use measuring tape to quantify the circumference of the muscle at a fixed distance from its insertion to note any differences.

It is important to observe the position of the patella in the seated position. If the patella is tilted laterally, giving it a "grasshopper-eye" appearance, this may indicate laterally directed forces on the patella. Patellar height may be best observed from the side. Normally the proximal aspect of the patella should line up with the anterior cortex of the distal femur in a seated position. An abnormally low patella, or patella baja, may represent a quadriceps tendon rupture. An abnormally high patella, or patella alta, will have an anterior tilt to the patella and can represent a patellar tendon rupture. In addition, patients with congenital patella alta may be at increased risk of patellar subluxation, owing to the increased time necessary for the patella to engage with the trochlea in knee flexion. The angle between the tibial tubercle and the patella (bent knee Q-angle) should also be observed. In normal individuals this angle averages 4°, but larger angles suggest external tibial torsion, which can contribute to patellar maltracking.[16] The best way to document abnormal lateralization of the tibial tubercle is not on clinical examination but rather by assessing the tibial tubercle/trochlear groove offset on a computed tomography scan.

Box 1
Beighton criteria

1. Rest palms of hands flat on floor with forward flexion of trunk with knees fully extended

2. Passive dorsiflexion of small fingers beyond 90°

3. Passive apposition of thumbs to volar aspects of forearm

4. Hyperextension of elbows beyond 10°

5. Hyperextension of knee beyond 10°

One point is awarded for each side of maneuvers 2 through 5 for a maximum total of 9 points. A score of 4 or more is consistent with joint hypermobility.

During the next step of the physical examination, passive and active range of motion of the knee should be measured and compared with that on the contralateral side. A decrease in active extension when compared with passive extension, also known as an extensor lag, may represent disruption of the extensor mechanism or motor weakness. Often any significant injury to the knee may cause a decrease in active extension secondary to pain. In this situation, an intra-articular anesthetic injection may assist in clarifying the true cause of lack of full active extension. A decrease in passive range of motion may be related to an intra-articular abnormality or may be due to tightness of any one of the muscle groups that cross the knee joint. Most of the individual muscle tightness is tested during the supine portion of the examination; however, tightness of the gastrocnemius muscle can be assessed at this point using the Silfverskiöld test. A positive test consists of tightness in ankle dorsiflexion with the knee extended that resolves when the knee is flexed.

During active range of motion, the patella should again be observed for any sudden lateral movement as it exits the trochlea, also known as the J-sign. It is suggested that the examiner place a hand over the patella during active range of motion to assess for patellofemoral crepitus or a grinding sensation. Johnson and colleagues[16] found that 40% of asymptomatic female patients had patellofemoral crepitus with range of motion. This examination finding is thus most specific when the crepitus is new, painful, and asymmetric. Quadriceps and hamstring strength may be tested by having the patient extend and flex the knee against resistance, and this should be compared with the contralateral side.

SUPINE

The greater part of the physical examination of the patellofemoral joint is performed with the patient in the supine position. First, the knee is assessed for any effusion to rule out any intra-articular process. A large swelling in the suprapatellar pouch is typical with large effusions, but may be more difficult to detect in the setting of smaller effusions or larger individuals. To test for an effusion in these situations, the examiner can push on any suspected swelling laterally or medially so that a transfer of the fluid can be observed on the opposite side of the knee. For subtle effusions, fluid can be "milked" both proximally and distally, and subtle bulging medially and laterally can be seen.

Palpation of the knee may be the most reliable examination maneuver to localize the source of any anterior knee pain (**Fig. 2**). The entire extensor mechanism is first palpated from proximal to distal. Initially the quadriceps tendon and its insertion at the superior aspect of the patella are palpated. Tenderness may represent quadriceps tendinopathy. Although rare, tenderness specifically at the superior pole of the patella may represent an osteochondrosis. Any gap felt while palpating the quadriceps tendon is suspicious for a tendon rupture. The patella is palpated next. Tenderness on the patella may represent a patella fracture or a symptomatic bipartite patella.

Next, the patella tendon and its insertion at the inferior pole are palpated. To improve palpation of the inferior pole of the patella, the examiner should initially press posteriorly on the superior pole of the patella, thus tilting the inferior pole anteriorly, making it easier to palpate. Tenderness, swelling, and warmth in this area are symptoms suggestive of patellar tendinopathy, also known as jumper's knee. Tenderness at the inferior pole of the patella in children may represent an osteochondrosis known as Sinding-Larsen-Johansson disease. A gap felt over the patellar tendon is suggestive of a tendon rupture. Tenderness or swelling along the patellar tendon would be significant for patellar tendinopathy or inflammation of the prepatellar bursa. The tibial

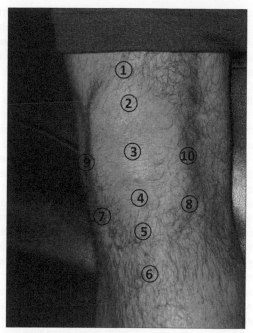

Fig. 2. Key points of palpation around the knee include (1) quadriceps tendon, (2) superior pole of patella, (3) patellar body, (4) inferior pole of patella, (5) patellar tendon, (6) tibial tubercle, (7) medial joint line, (8) lateral joint line, (9) medial retinaculum, and (10) lateral retinaculum.

tubercle is then palpated, and any tenderness and prominence noted there in a skeletally immature subject may be suggestive of tibial tubercle apophysitis, known as Osgood-Schlatter disease. In a mature patient, pain over the tibial tubercle may represent bursitis or a remnant ossicle from Osgood-Schlatter disease as a child.

The anterior joint line is then palpated. First, the fat pad of Hoffa is felt by palpating just medial and lateral the patellar tendon. Tenderness here may be secondary to inflammation of the fat pad. The medial and lateral retinacula are then palpated. Tenderness over the lateral retinaculum has been found in patients with chronic patellar malalignment.[11,17] Tenderness along the medial retinaculum, specifically along the medial patellofemoral ligament (MPFL) and its insertions, are often found in patellar dislocations. Though not as sensitive, a defect in the medial retinaculum may sometimes be felt. The medial synovial plica can then be palpated by rolling one's fingers over the plica fold located between the medial patella and adductor tubercle of the femur. Reproduction of pain with this maneuver is consistent with irritation of the medial plica. Pain in the medial plica is also often exacerbated when performing a lateral McMurray maneuver, whereas it is relieved or less affected by a medial McMurray maneuver.

The medial and lateral articular surfaces of the patella can be palpated by tilting the patella and curling one's fingers around each facet. Tenderness can represent an articular injury; however, as retropatellar palpation can be painful in normal individuals, the contralateral side should be palpated for comparison.

It is also important to palpate other structures around the knee that present in similar fashion to patellofemoral problems and may produce anterior knee pain. Conditions such as pes anserine bursitis, iliotibial band tendinopathy, meniscal tears, and physeal injuries in children can be assessed by palpation of the pes anserine insertion, Gerdy tubercle, the medial and lateral joint lines, and the distal femoral physis, respectively.

After palpating all relevant structures, patellofemoral-specific maneuvers that target specific diagnoses should be undertaken. It is best to group these together into diagnostic series for the key diagnoses of instability, arthroses, and tendinopathy with motor unit tightness.

Regarding instability, the patellar glide and apprehension tests are performed by grasping the patella with the knee flexed to 20° and translating it medially and laterally. It must be borne in mind that 95% of patellar instability goes laterally, and that medial instability usually has an iatrogenic component. Medial glide of less than 1 quadrant of the patellar width is consistent with lateral tightness, whereas glide of 3 quadrants or more in either direction is consistent with hypermobility of the patella (**Fig. 3**). Tanner and colleagues[18] has shown that lateral displacement of the distal patella during a glide test is more sensitive than direct lateral displacement for detecting MPFL injuries. If the patient experiences apprehension and a sense of impending dislocation with lateral translation, a positive apprehension test and patellar instability are indicated.

Another method for evaluating patellofemoral tightness is with the patellar tilt test. In this examination the physician presses posteriorly on the medial aspect of the patella with the knee extended, causing the lateral portion of the patella to move anteriorly. If the lateral patella does not move past horizontal, this suggests lateral tightness. It is an important test because it is the only validated indication for performing a lateral release for patellofemoral pain. This examination can then be performed on the medial side as well, looking for excessive medial retinacular tightness.

Regarding patellofemoral chondrosis, the compression test is useful for assessing chondral injuries as a result of arthritis or a previous patellar dislocation. This test is

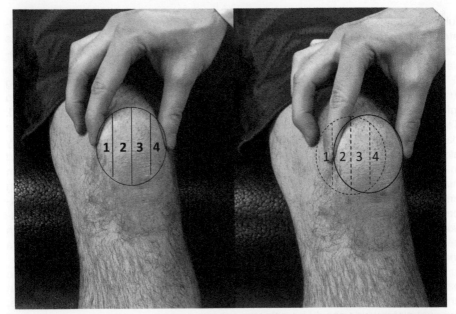

Fig. 3. The patellar glide test is performed by grasping the patella with the knee flexed to 20° and translating it medially and laterally. Medial glide of less than 1 quadrant of the patellar width is consistent with lateral tightness, whereas glide of 3 quadrants or more in either direction is consistent with hypermobility (The *numbers* represent quadrants of patella).

performed by directly pressing on the patella as the knee is flexed. Increased pain indicates a positive test, and the degree of flexion at which pain is greatest can help localize which part of the patella or trochlea is affected. Because lateral patella dislocations are often associated with medial facet articular damage, the authors have found that decompressing the affected lesion by holding the patella medially or laterally during range of motion can also be a valuable clue as to whether realignment procedures will be beneficial. A variation of this test can be performed with the patient supine with the knee relaxed and in full extension. The examiner resists proximal migration of the patella while the patient is asked to fire the quadriceps muscle. Increased pain directly beneath the patella once again confirms the likely diagnosis of patellofemoral arthrosis.

A thorough patellofemoral examination is completed by evaluating the tightness of the muscles crossing the knee, as they can increase stresses across the patellofemoral joint and contribute to patellofemoral abnormalities. Determination of tight muscle groups can ultimately help to direct physical therapy. The popliteal angle is measured to evaluate hamstring tightness. The hip is flexed to 90° and the knee is passively extended as far as possible, and the knee angle is then measured. Quadriceps tendon tightness is assessed with the patient in a prone position while hyperflexing the knee. Iliopsoas and rectus femoris tightness are assessed with the modified Thomas test. In this test, the patient lies supine with the legs first lying over end of the table. Both hips are flexed up to the patient's chest, and the patient grabs on the nontested limb with both hands. The examiner stabilizes this leg while the patient extends the tested hip with the knee flexed. An inability for that limb to reach horizontal represents either a tight iliopsoas or rectus. If the tightness resolves when the knee is extended, this localizes the tightness to the rectus. While in this position it is also useful to test for any pain with range of motion of the hip, as pain originating from the hip may be referred to the knee. For evaluating tightness of the iliotibial band (ITB), an Ober test is performed with the patient lying on the unaffected side. With the knee flexed and the hip extended, the upper leg is brought into adduction with the tester preventing any hip rotation. A patient with a tight ITB will have difficulty adducting the leg past horizontal. Ultimately, a complete examination of flexibility around the hip and knee will optimize a targeted rehabilitation plan and improve outcomes of most patellofemoral problems.

SUMMARY

Examination of the patellofemoral joint can prove to be challenging. Although certain acute injuries such as patella fracture or tendon rupture can be diagnosed quickly, more chronic injuries such as patellar subluxation and patellofemoral pain syndrome are more difficult to diagnose because of the subtlety of the examination findings. The source of the problem can also vary, and must be identified to direct treatment. Adding to the complexity is that other structures around the knee may present with anterior knee pain and can be mistaken for patellofemoral disorder, which is why the patellofemoral examination should be performed in the context of a complete knee examination. For all of these reasons, performing a thorough and systematic examination of the patellofemoral joint can lead to optimal outcomes for patients.

REFERENCES

1. Earl JE, Vetter CS. Patellofemoral pain. Phys Med Rehabil Clin N Am 2007;18: 439–58.

2. Messier SP, Davis SE, Curl WW, et al. Etiologic factors associated with patellofemoral pain in runners. Med Sci Sports Exerc 1991;9:1008–15.
3. Post WR. Clinical evaluation of patients with patellofemoral disorders. Arthroscopy 1999;15:841–51.
4. Ireland M, Willson J, Ballantyne B, et al. Hip strength in females with and without patellofemoral pain. J Orthop Sports Phys Ther 2003;33:671–6.
5. Powers C. The influence of altered lower-extremity kinematics on patellofemoral joint dysfunction: a theoretical perspective. J Orthop Sports Phys Ther 2003;33:639–46.
6. Riegger-Krugh C, Keysor J. Skeletal malalignments of the lower quarter: correlated and compensatory motions and postures. J Orthop Sports Phys Ther 1996;2:164–70.
7. Prins MR, van der Wurff P. Females with patellofemoral pain syndrome have weak hip muscles: a systematic review. Aust J Physiother 2009;55:9–15.
8. White LC, Dolphin P, Dixon J. Hamstring length in patellofemoral pain syndrome. Physiotherapy 2009;95:24–8.
9. Witvrouw E, Lysens R, Bellemans J, et al. Intrinsic risk factors for the development of anterior knee pain in an athletic population. A two-year prospective study. Am J Sports Med 2000;28:480–9.
10. Smith AD, Stroud L, McQueen C. Flexibility and anterior knee pain in adolescent elite figure skaters. J Pediatr Orthop 1991;11:77–82.
11. Fulkerson JP, Kalenak A, Rosenberg TD, et al. Patellofemoral pain. Instr Course Lect 1994;41:57–71.
12. Al-Rawi Z, Nessan AH. Joint hypermobility in patients with chondromalacia patellae. Br J Rheumatol 1997;36:1324–7.
13. Barber Foss KD, Ford KR, Myer GD, et al. Generalized Joint laxity associated with increased medial foot loading in female athletes. J Athl Train 2009;44:356–62.
14. Bose K, Kanagasuntherum R, Osman M. Vastus medialis oblique: an anatomical and physiologic study. Orthopedics 1980;3:880–3.
15. Witvrouw E, Lysens R, Bellemans J, et al. Open versus closed kinetic chain exercises for patellofemoral pain. A prospective, randomized study. Am J Sports Med 2000;28:687–94.
16. Johnson LL, van Dyk GE, Green JR 3rd, et al. Clinical assessment of asymptomatic knees: comparison of men and women. Arthroscopy 1998;4:347–59.
17. Merchant AC. Patellofemoral malalignment and instabilities. In: Ewing JW, editor. Articular cartilage and knee joint function: basic science and arthroscopy. New York: Raven Press Ltd; 1990. p. 79–91.
18. Tanner SM, Garth WP Jr, Soileau R, et al. A modified test for patellar instability: the biomechanical basis. Clin J Sport Med 2003;13:327–38.

Imaging of the Patellofemoral Joint

Stephen Thomas, MD, David Rupiper, MD, G. Scott Stacy, MD*

KEYWORDS

- Magnetic resonance imaging • Patellofemoral joint • Patellar instability
- Patellar malalignment

KEY POINTS

- The patellofemoral (PF) joint is a complex articulation, with interplay between the osseous and soft tissue structures to maintain the balance between knee mobility and stability.
- Disorders of the PF joint can be a source of anterior knee pain.
- Imaging of the knee is important for evaluating patients with knee pain.

INTRODUCTION

The patellofemoral (PF) joint is a complex articulation, dependent on both dynamic and static restraints for its function and stability. Disease in the PF articulation is implicated in anterior knee pain (AKP), which has a reported prevalence affecting between 20% and 40% of the adolescent population, with a higher prevalence in athletes.[1] AKP is a common symptom and accounts for up to 10% of all visits to orthopedic and musculoskeletal clinics.[2] The biomechanics of the PF joint are complex, because it transmits tensile force from the quadriceps to the patellar tendon. The patella centralizes the divergent forces of the quadriceps muscles and transmits the tension around the femur to the patellar tendon. The patella increases the mechanical advantage of the extensor muscles by increasing the knee extension moment arm through the entire range of knee motion.[3] Imaging of the knee is important for evaluating patients with knee pain.

IMAGING OF THE KNEE
Radiographs

Conventional radiography is commonly the first imaging modality in evaluating knee pain. A standard radiographic examination of the knee includes frontal, lateral, and axial views. Frontal views are usually obtained as anterior-posterior projections, with or without weight bearing, and are the least useful view for evaluating the patella.

Department of Radiology, University of Chicago, 5841 South Maryland Avenue, MC 2026, Chicago, IL 60637, USA
* Corresponding author.
E-mail address: sstacy@radiology.bsd.uchicago.edu

Clin Sports Med 33 (2014) 413–436
http://dx.doi.org/10.1016/j.csm.2014.03.007
0278-5919/14/$ – see front matter © 2014 Elsevier Inc. All rights reserved.

sportsmed.theclinics.com

Lateral views are usually obtained in mild flexion (approximately 30°) in a lateral recumbent position, but may be obtained cross-table especially in the setting of trauma. Axial/tangential views (often generically referred to as sunrise views) are obtained to evaluate the PF articulation, including the morphology of the patella, size of the patella with respect to the trochlea, and sulcus angle. There are several positioning methods to obtain the axial images. One common method is the Merchant view, which is a superior-to-inferior projection obtained with the patient's knees flexed 45° over the edge of the table and the beam angled 30° to the femora.[4] The Laurin technique is an axial image obtained with the beam projection from inferior to superior and the knee in 20° of flexion; it is considered more sensitive for patella subluxation, which occurs between 20° and 30° of flexion.[5]

Magnetic Resonance Imaging

Magnetic resonance imaging (MRI), with its superior soft tissue contrast resolution and multiplanar capability, is an excellent modality to view the PF joint. Imaging is performed using a dedicated multichannel knee coil, preferably on a high field unit (≥1.5 T). Standard sequences should include a fat-suppressed sequence, which improves conspicuity for marrow edema patterns and fluid collections by allowing better use of the full dynamic range of the gray scale.[6]

An intermediate echo-time two-dimensional (2D) non–fat-suppressed fast/turbo spin-echo image provides good differential contrast between the intermediate signal intensity of articular cartilage, the low signal intensity of fibrocartilage, and the high signal intensity of synovial fluid and allows imaging of the grayscale stratification of cartilage (**Fig. 1**), which corresponds to cartilage zonal anatomy.[7] Newer three-dimensional (3D) fast spin-echo techniques or fat-suppressed T1-weighted

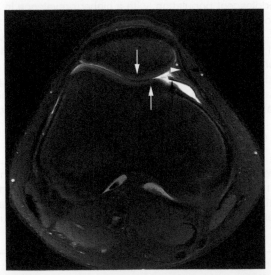

Fig. 1. Fat-suppressed proton-density-weighted transverse MRI of the knee shows normal patellar and trochlear cartilage (*white arrows*). Note the grayscale stratification of the cartilage with lower signal intensity in the radial zone (close to the bone) and the higher signal intensity in the transitional zone (closer to the surface). Note also the distal portion of the medial patellofemoral ligament (*white arrowhead*), tendinous fibers of the vastus medialis obliquus (*black arrowhead*), and mediopatellar plica (*black arrow*).

gradient-echo sequences allow quantitative automated or semiautomated techniques for cartilage imaging.[8]

ANATOMY
Patellar Anatomy and Variants

The patella is the largest sesamoid bone in the human body. Seven facets located in the proximal two-thirds of the patella form the articular surface of the patella. The odd facet located in the medial patella engages the medial femoral condyle as the patella rotates in knee flexion greater than 90°. The distal pole of the patella attaches to the proximal patellar tendon to transmit the force from the quadriceps to the tibia.[9]

Patellar facet size is variable, but generally, the lateral facet is longer than the medial facet in approximately two-thirds of people, as seen on axial imaging. The Wiberg[10] classification scheme is used to describe the different medial and lateral patellar facet sizes. The Wiberg type I patella (with a prevalence of 10%) has nearly equal-sized medial and lateral facets. The Wiberg type II patella is the most common type, with a prevalence of 65%; the medial facet is either flat or mildly convex. The Wiberg type III patella is the second most common morphology, seen in 25% of cases, with a smaller convex medial facet.[9]

Many patellar anatomic variants have been described. Variants in size include patella magna and patella parva. Shape variants include hunter cap, half-moon, pebble, and Baumgartl, with a protuberant medial facet as a Wiberg type III variant.[9] Aplastic, hypoplastic, bipartite or multipartite, and duplicated patellae are other variants.

Bipartite Patella

Bipartite patella is a common radiologic finding, seen in approximately 2% of individuals, and represents failed fusion of a secondary ossification center with the body of the patella. It can be bilateral in 40% of the cases and is 9 times more common in males. Three types have been described. Type I involves the inferior pole of the patella, type II involves the lateral margin, and type III is the most common, involving the superolateral aspect at the insertion of the vastus lateralis muscle.[11] In most patients, bipartite patella is an incidental finding in which the morphologically segmented patella remains asymptomatic and the associated articular cartilage remains intact. In response to overuse or acute injury, the synchondrosis may become either partly or completely disrupted, allowing abnormal motion, friction, and subsequently, the development of edema (**Fig. 2**).[12]

Dorsal Defect of the Patella

Dorsal defect of the patella is a well-defined benign subchondral lesion in the superolateral aspect of the patella, occurring in approximately 1% of the population. The lesion presents with a characteristic radiographic appearance consisting of a rounded focus of radiolucency surrounded by a sclerotic margin and can vary in diameter from 4 mm to 26 mm. On MRI, the overlying articular cartilage appears intact and can be thickened to fill the subchondral defect (**Fig. 3**).[11]

Patellar Cartilage

Patellar cartilage can be accurately evaluated with MRI, with better performance on high field units. Morphologic and subchondral disease can be imaged with 2D proton-density-weighted, intermediate-weighted, and T2-weighted fast spin-echo sequences, 3D spoiled gradient-echo or fast low-angle shot gradient-echo sequences, and dual-echo steady-state sequences.[13] Patellar cartilage is thicker than articular cartilage in most other joints, measuring 4 to 5 mm.[14]

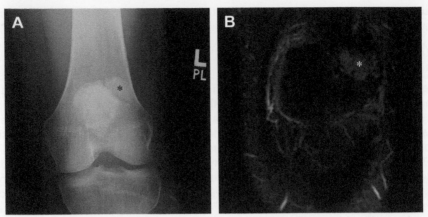

Fig. 2. Bipartite patella. (*A*) Anteroposterior knee radiograph shows an unfused ossification center along the superolateral aspect of the patella (*asterisk*). (*B*) Fat-suppressed T2-weighted coronal MRI of the patella shows edema within the unfused ossification center (*asterisk*). Such edema may be associated with pain in patients with a bipartite patella.

Trochlea

The trochlea is formed from the medial and lateral facets of the femoral sulcus. The cartilaginous surface of the patellar groove forms a tunnellike track for the patella to move during knee flexion. The condyles help stabilize the patella, preventing lateral translation.[14] The trochlea deepens from its proximal to distal aspect.[9] The femoral trochlear facet cartilage is either equal to or thinner than the patellar cartilage by 2 to 3 mm. The cartilage is thinner on the medial trochlear facet than the lateral trochlear facet. The lateral trochlear cartilage layer extends more proximally than the medial trochlear cartilage layer.[15]

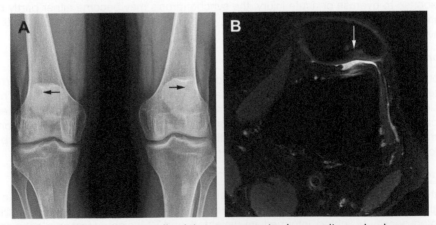

Fig. 3. Dorsal defect of the patella. (*A*) Anteroposterior knee radiographs show a small round lucency (*arrows*) within the superolateral aspect of the left and right patellae. (*B*) Fat-suppressed proton-density-weighted transverse MRI of the knee shows the defect (*arrow*) filled with cartilage.

Quadriceps Tendon

The quadriceps tendon is the common tendon formed between the myofascial junctions of the superficial layer of the rectus femoris muscle, the middle layers of the vastus medialis and vastus lateralis muscles, and the deep layer of the vastus intermedius muscle. On sagittal and axial non–fat-suppressed spin-echo sequences, the normal quadriceps tendon has a variable laminar appearance. The tendinous contributions from each muscle can be identified as 4 separate layers (6%); as fusion of the components from the vastus medialis and lateralis muscle to form the middle layer, resulting in 3 bands (56%); as fusion of the anterior and middle layer(s) to form 2 bands with the deep layer (30%); or as fusion of all layers to form 1 band (8%).[16] The layers converge at the broad insertion of the quadriceps tendon on the patella (**Fig. 4**). The most anterior fibers of the quadriceps tendon, the contribution from the rectus femoris, blend over the anterior aspect of the patella, forming an aponeurosis connecting to the patellar tendon, providing structural components of the vertical and horizontal tensile bracing system. Biomechanically, the quadriceps tendon and the patella are integral parts of the active and passive extensor mechanisms of the knee joint.[17]

Patellar Tendon

The patellar tendon is the continuation of the quadriceps tendon, composed mostly of the rectus femoris component passing over the anterior aspect of the patella, and inserts on the tibial tubercle (see **Fig. 4**). The patellar tendon is the primary restraint in the coronal plane, limiting patellar movement proximally to 10 mm.[18] The normal anteroposterior thickness of the patellar tendon is less than that of the quadriceps tendon.[18]

Medial Patellar Soft Tissue Restraints

Medial soft tissue restraints attaching to the patella are crucial to prevent lateral patellar dislocation as forces are transferred through the extensor mechanism. There is considerable variability in the literature of the description of the medial supporting

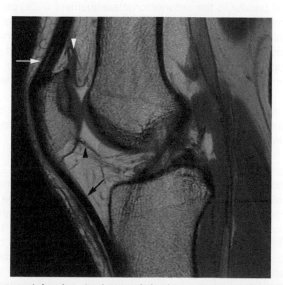

Fig. 4. Intermediate-weighted sagittal MRI of the knee shows normal striated appearance of quadriceps tendon (*white arrow*), normal patellar tendon (*black arrow*), and portions of the suprapatellar plica (*white arrowhead*) and infrapatellar plica (*black arrowhead*).

structures of the knee, and a detailed discussion is beyond the scope of this article. The Warren and Marshall model describes a 3-layer concept of patellar support in the medial aspect of the knee. The superficial layer (layer I) includes the crural fascia. The intermediate layer (layer II) includes the superficial portion of the medial collateral ligament (MCL), as well as the medial patellofemoral ligament (MPFL), which extends in a fan-shaped manner from the medial patellar edge to the femur along the medial epicondyle and is an important medial static ligamentous restraint. The patellar attachment of the MPFL blends with the medial patellar retinaculum as it attaches to the patellar edge. The deep layer (layer III) is formed by the joint capsule and deep portion of the MCL.[19]

The medial patellar retinaculum and MPFL are best imaged with axial and coronal T2-weighted fast spin-echo or gradient-echo pulse sequences at MRI (see **Fig. 1**). The patellar third of the MPFL blends with the vastus medialis obliquus muscle, which results in a broader attachment and greater conspicuity at MRI. The femoral third of the ligament is thin and may not be depicted well.[20] The vastus medialis obliquus, which arises from the medial part of the femur and attaches to the proximal portion of the patella, is considered a primary dynamic restraint.[21]

Synovial Plicae of the Knee

The knee joint is believed to be composed of 3 compartments (medial, lateral, and suprapatellar), which are partitioned by synovial septa. The synovial plicae are normal structures that are formed from folds of synovial tissue and are considered remnants of synovial membranes.[22]

The suprapatellar plica runs obliquely downward from the synovium at the anterior aspect of the femoral metaphysis to the posterior aspect of the quadriceps tendon, inserting above the patella (see **Fig. 4**). It may impinge on cartilage of the superomedial angle of the trochlea in flexion.[22]

The infrapatellar plica is the most common plica in the knee. It can be easily identified at MRI as a linear low signal intensity structure running from the intercondylar notch anterior and parallel to the anterior cruciate ligament (ACL) on sagittal images through the Hoffa fat pad, which inserts on the inferior pole of the patella (see **Fig. 4**).[23]

The mediopatellar plica arises from the medial wall of the knee joint, runs obliquely downward, and inserts into the synovium covering the infrapatellar fat pad (see **Fig. 1**). When the mediopatellar plica covers the anterior surface of the medial femoral condyle, it can impinge between the condyle and the patella, thereby becoming symptomatic.[24]

The lateral patellar plica is the least common plica of the knee. It originates in the lateral wall above the popliteus hiatus and attaches to the infrapatellar fat pad. If present, it is very thin, and located 1 to 2 cm lateral to the patella.[22]

Patellar Tilt

Patellar tilt is defined as the angle subtended by a line joining the medial and lateral edges of the patella and the horizontal. Abnormal patellar tilt may be present with or without patellar translation. Abnormal lateral tilt is more frequently symptomatic than mere subluxation. Abnormal patellar tilt was formerly believed to be one of the leading factors causing dislocations, caused by vastus medialis obliquus insufficiency. However, it seems to be the result of a complex interplay of factors, including trochlear and patellar shape and congruence, as well as medial restraint insufficiency.[25] Abnormal lateral tilt can be associated with patellar maltracking, previous dislocation, or excessive lateral pressure syndrome, and can be caused by a tight lateral retinaculum.[21]

Axial radiograph

The lateral PF angle is formed between a line along the lateral patellar facet and a line across the anterior condylar margins; normally this angle is more than 8° and open laterally, with parallel lines or a medially opening angle representing lateral patellar tilt, which is nonspecific but can be an indirect sign of previous dislocation (**Fig. 5**).[14,25]

The PF index is the ratio (M/L) between the thickness of the medial joint space (M) and the lateral joint space (L). Normally, it measures 1.6 or less. A ratio of greater than 1.6 is abnormal and indicates lateral patellar tilt (see **Fig. 5**).[25]

Lateral radiograph

Well-positioned lateral radiographs on which the posterior aspects of the medial and lateral femoral condyles overlap should show the median ridge of the patella as the most posterior structure, with the more anterior line formed by the lateral facet.

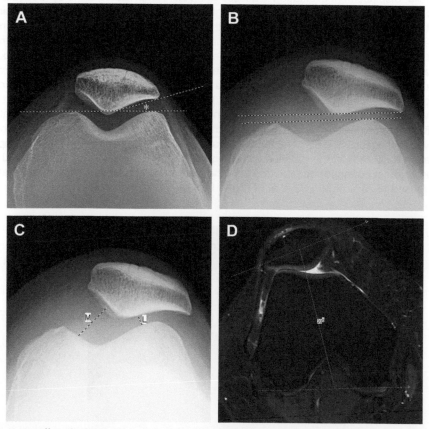

Fig. 5. Patellar tilt. (*A*) Axial radiograph of the knee shows normal lateral PF angle (*asterisk*) opening laterally. (*B*) Axial radiograph of the knee of a different patient shows parallel lines along the lateral patellar facet and along the anterior condylar margins, indicating lateral patellar tilt. (*C*) Axial radiograph of the same patient as in (*B*) shows widened medial joint space (M) relative to the lateral joint space (L), resulting in a high PF index, indicating lateral patellar tilt. (*D*) Fat-suppressed proton-density transverse MRI of the knee shows lateral patellar tilt with an angle of 20° (normal<10°) between the axis of the patella and a line tangent to the femoral condyles posteriorly.

With progressive lateral patellar tilt, these structures are superimposed, and then, this relationship is reversed, with the median ridge seen as the more anterior structure.[14]

MRI

Quantification of patellar tilt angle can be performed on an axial MRI of the knee in a manner similar to that using radiographs. Alternatively, the angle between the line joining the medial and lateral borders of the patella at the patellar midpoint (axis of the patella) and the line tangent to the posterior femoral condyles can be used to quantify patellar tilt; it is more analogous to the clinical examination (see **Fig. 5**).[21] Patients with an MRI tilt angle of 10° or greater correlate with significant tilt on physical examination, whereas a tilt angle of less than 10° was associated with the absence of significant tilt on physical examination.[25]

Patellar Displacement (Subluxation)

Patellar displacement evaluation is assessed on axial knee radiographs by measuring the congruence angle. First, the sulcus angle, formed by lines from the deepest point of the intercondylar sulcus connected to the most anterior points of the medial and lateral condyles, is measured. Two other lines are drawn from its vertex: one bisecting the sulcus angle (reference line) and another to the apex of the patella. The angle between these 2 lines is the congruence angle, which is considered positive if the line to the patellar apex is situated lateral to the reference line. The average congruence angle is –6° (standard deviation [SD] ± 11°) (**Fig. 6**).[25]

MRI does not accurately assess PF alignment, because MRI of the knee is usually performed in extension. When evaluating patellar subluxation by computed tomography (CT) images at 30°, 60°, and 90° of flexion in normal knees and with the quadriceps relaxed, only 13% of the patellae were centered in the trochlea in full extension (the median crest corresponded exactly with the intercondylar groove), whereas this rate increased to 29% at 30°, 63% at 60°, and 96% at 90° of flexion.[26]

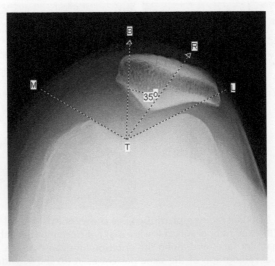

Fig. 6. Patellar subluxation. Axial radiograph of the knee shows the sulcus angle (MTL) bisected by line BT. The congruence angle is formed between line BT and line RT extending from the patellar apex to the deepest point of the intercondylar sulcus (trochlea). The congruence angle of +35° in this patient indicates lateral subluxation (normal average –6°).

Patellar Height

Patella alta is defined as a high-riding patella in relation to the femoral trochlea, caused by an effectively lengthened patellar tendon (**Fig. 7**). The patella requires higher degrees of knee flexion (in normal patients, patellar engagement occurs around 20° of flexion) to engage the trochlea, which reduces contact and stability with shallow flexion.[27] Patella alta is usually an asymptomatic normal variant but also increases the risk of future patellar dislocation caused by altered mechanics. Patella alta can be present with patellar tendon ruptures and is present in approximately 25% of acute patellar dislocations as evidence of previous injury.[20]

Patellar height can be measured radiographically using a variety of methods on the lateral radiograph. The 4 most widely used and studied methods include those described by Insall-Salvati, Grelsamer-Meadows (modified Insall-Salvati), Blackburne-Peel, and Caton-Deschamps. Controversy remains over which radiographic method is best, but many argue that the Caton and Blackburne methods are the most accurate and reproducible.[28]

The Insall-Salvati method seems to be most widely used, because it is the historic standard and is simple; the normal values are easy to remember (0.8–1.2), and the calculation simply compares the ratio between the length of the patellar tendon and the longest sagittal length of the patella. Measurement is made on a lateral radiograph in 20° to 70° of flexion. Insall determined that this ratio is normally 1. A ratio less than 0.8 indicates a patella baja and greater than 1.2 patella alta. Limitations to this method include variations in osseous patellar morphology and osseous hypertrophy of the patella at its superior or inferior margins, making accurate patellar length measurements difficult.[28]

The other 3 methods do not use osseous patellar length in the equation, but instead use patellar articular surface (PAS) length; however, identification of patellar articular margins on radiographs can be difficult.

The Grelsamer-Meadows or modified Insall-Salvati method is a ratio of (1) the distance between the inferior PAS and the patellar tendon insertion on the tibial tubercle

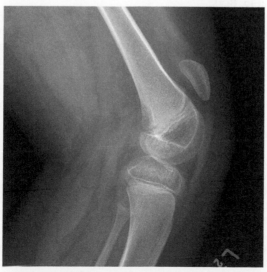

Fig. 7. Patella alta. Lateral radiograph of the knee shows high-riding patella, indicating patella alta.

to (2) the length of the PAS as measured on a lateral radiograph in 20° to 70° of flexion. Patella alta is diagnosed when the ratio is greater than 2.[28]

The Blackburne-Peel and Caton-Deschamps methods use a different inferior landmark, replacing the need for identification of the tibial tubercle. The Blackburne-Peel method uses an anterior horizontal line projected across the tibial plateau. The normal ratio of (1) the distance from the horizontal line to the inferior edge of the PAS to (2) the length of the PAS should be between 0.8 and 1.0.[28]

The Caton-Deschamps method uses the anterosuperior angle of the tibial plateau as the inferior reference point. The ratio of (1) the distance between the inferior edge of the PAS to the anterosuperior angle of the tibial plateau to (2) the length of the PAS should be between 0.6 and 1.3.[28]

MRI

Although these measurements were created using radiographic evaluations, these techniques can be translated to MR measurements of the patellar height ratio as assessed on sagittal intermediate-weighted sequences.[20] The cutoff values for patella alta and baja derived from radiographs many not be directly applicable to MRI. For the Blackburne-Peel ratio, an additional adjustment of 0.09 is needed between radiographs and MRI.[29]

When comparing the MRI criteria for patella alta and baja as measured by the Insall-Salvati method on sagittal MR sequences, it was found to be 1.50 and less than 0.74, respectively.[30]

APOPHYSITIS

Sinding-Larsen-Johansson syndrome is a form of traction apophysitis (chronic repetitive microtrauma) at the inferior pole of the patella at the patellar tendon insertion. This syndrome is similar to but less common than Osgood-Schlatter disease (OSD) at the tibial tubercle. MRI findings include thickening of the proximal patellar tendon, with marrow edema at the proximal pole of the patella extending into the adjacent fat. Radiographs may show patella alta and tiny osseous fragments adjacent to the inferior pole of the patella (**Fig. 8**).[27]

OSD is considered a form of traction apophysitis at the tibial tubercle. OSD is most common among adolescent male athletes in sports that require jumping and kicking and is bilateral in up to 50% of cases. MRI findings include thickening and edema of the distal patellar tendon, a fluid-distended deep infrapatellar bursa, edema of the surrounding soft tissue, and bone marrow edema subjacent to the tibial tubercle. Knee radiographs may show fragmentation of the tibial tubercle, soft tissue swelling, and obliteration of the inferior angle of the Hoffa fat pad (see **Fig. 8**).[27]

CHONDROMALACIA PATELLA AND OSTEOARTHRITIS

Chondromalacia patella, also known as runner's knee, is a term for patellar articular cartilage loss in the setting of AKP. Simple chondromalacia patella is common in adolescents and young adults, characterized by cartilage softening and fissuring (**Fig. 9**). The link between progression of chondromalacia patella to osteoarthritis is not clear. PF osteoarthritis is usually encountered in older individuals, and its cause is considered multifactorial.[27]

Radiographs are insensitive for early cartilage changes but can detect osteoarthritis in its later stages, as shown by joint space narrowing, osteophyte formation, subchondral sclerosis, subchondral cysts, or ossified loose joint bodies. MRI most accurately depicts cartilage abnormalities with a 4-stage grading system designed

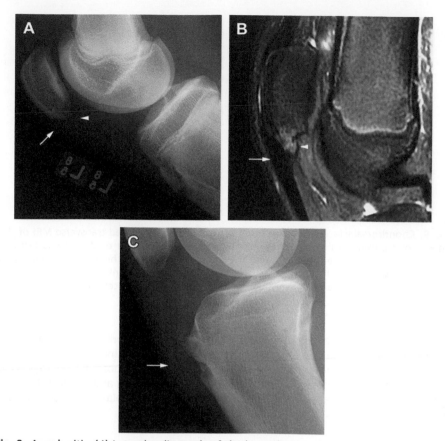

Fig. 8. Apophysitis. (A) Lateral radiograph of the knee shows mild thickening of the proximal patellar tendon (*arrow*) and ossific irregularity along the inferior margin of the patella (*arrowhead*) compatible with Sinding-Larsen-Johansson disease. (B) Fat-suppressed T2-weighted sagittal MRI of the knee of the same patient as in (A) shows thickening of patellar tendon (*arrow*) and edema in the irregular ossific protuberance projecting from inferior aspect of patella (*arrowhead*). (C) Lateral radiograph of the knee shows thickening of the distal patellar tendon (*arrow*) and fragmentation of the underlying tibial tubercle in this patient with Osgood-Schlatter disease.

to correspond to the Outerbridge grading system devised for arthroscopy. In general, MRI grading accuracy of PF cartilage lesions is excellent for high-grade lesions (>50% thickness) and clearly depicts underlying marrow signal abnormalities (**Fig. 10**); however, accuracy is variably diminished for low-grade lesions (<50% thickness) without underlying marrow signal abnormalities. Recent studies have indicated that PF articular cartilage grading by both MRI and arthroscopy may have poor correlation with symptoms.[27]

The cartilage black line sign or trochlear cleft is a rare MRI finding in young active individuals. It is seen as a linear T2 hypointense focus within and oriented perpendicular to the articular cartilage, typically centered in the trochlear trough, where it appears to extend through the entire thickness of the trochlear cartilage (**Fig. 11**). It most likely indicates an incomplete cartilage fissure, which may rarely progress to a full-thickness defect.[31]

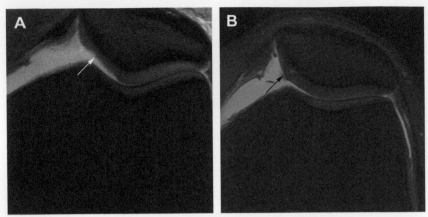

Fig. 9. Chondromalacia. (*A*) Fat-suppressed proton-density-weighted transverse MRI of the knee shows partial-thickness cartilage loss along the medial facet of the patella (*arrow*), with preservation of the cartilage along the lateral facet and trochlea. (*B*) Fat-suppressed proton-density-weighted transverse MRI of the knee of a different patient shows a full-thickness fissure of the articular cartilage of the medial patellar facet (*arrow*).

TROCHLEAR DYSPLASIA

Trochlear dysplasia is an important factor contributing to chronic PF instability. With trochlear dysplasia, the trochlear joint surface is flattened proximally, and the concavity is less pronounced distally. As a result, the femoral sulcus is not sufficient to provide the osseous restraint needed to prevent lateral patellar tracking and lateral dislocation of the patella at the initiation of flexion.[20] Signs of trochlear dysplasia are found in more than 85% of patients with patellar dislocation.[32]

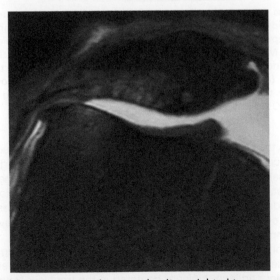

Fig. 10. Osteoarthritis. Fat-suppressed proton-density-weighted transverse MRI of the knee shows full-thickness cartilage loss along the lateral facet of the patella and femoral trochlea, with edemalike signal and cysts in the underlying subchondral marrow, as well as small osteophytes.

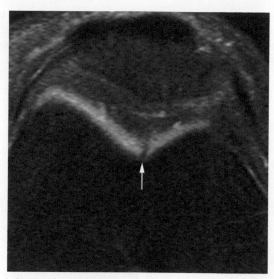

Fig. 11. Trochlear cleft. Fat-suppressed proton-density-weighted transverse MRI of the knee shows a thin linear band of low signal intensity (*arrow*) centrally within the femoral trochlea.

Radiographs are often used for initial evaluation of trochlear anatomy and the search for trochlear dysplasia. Strict lateral views, with perfect superimposition of the posterior aspects of the medial and lateral femoral condyles, can be used to evaluate trochlear dysplasia. The relationship of the anterior condylar borders with the intercondylar sulcus can be analyzed, although this is dependent on excellent positioning and degraded by even slight degrees of rotation. A measurable depth of 5 mm should be present, and anything less suggests instability risk.[14]

The crossing sign is a line represented by the deepest part of the trochlear groove crossing the anterior aspect of the condyles; it marks the point at which the trochlea becomes flat. The double contour sign is a double line at the anterior aspect of the condyles and is present if the medial condyle is hypoplastic, with its anterior margin projecting posterior to that of the lateral condyle. The supratrochlear spur is found in the superolateral aspect of the trochlea and represents the global prominence of the trochlea (**Fig. 12**).[25,32]

Axial radiographs are useful for measurement of the sulcus angle, which is formed by lines from the deepest point of the intercondylar sulcus connected to the anterior tips of each femoral condyle. The normal mean value is 138° (SD ± 6). Angles greater than 150° are found in trochlear dysplasia. The sulcus angle measurement is impossible in flat or convex trochleae. An important issue when obtaining axial views is that radiographs obtained with higher flexion angles show the lower part of the trochlea, frequently missing the dysplasia present in its upper portion. For this reason, a 20° to 45° flexion view is preferred.[20,25]

Based on these criteria, Dejour and colleagues[32] proposed a 4-category system to classify trochlear dysplasia:

Type A: normal shape of the trochlea preserved but a shallow trochlear groove on axial views. The crossing sign is the only sign present on the lateral view.
Type B: markedly flattened or even convex trochlea on the axial view. The crossing sign and the supratrochlear spur are present on the lateral view.

Type C: asymmetric trochlear facets, with the lateral facet being too high and the medial facet being hypoplastic, which results in the flattened joint surface forming an oblique plane. On the lateral view, the crossing sign and the double contour sign are present, but there is no spur.

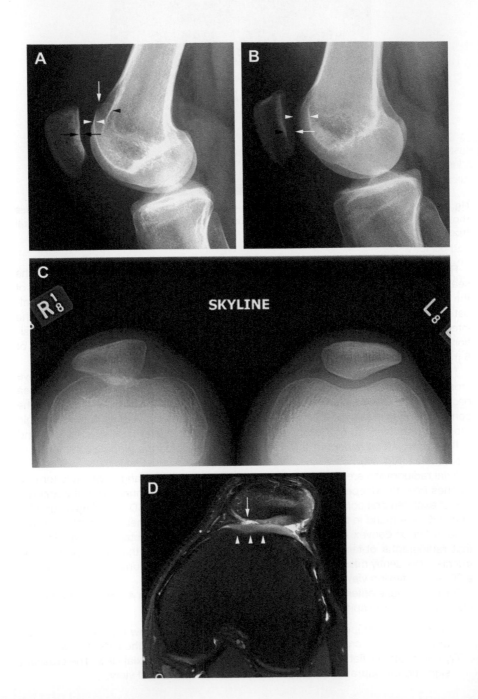

Type D: in addition to the features of type C, a vertical link between medial and lateral facets (cliff pattern on parasagittal images) is present. On the lateral view the crossing sign, supratrochlear spur, and double contour are present.[20,25]

Axial/sagittal MR images allow accurate identification of the type of trochlear anomaly. MRI has been shown to allow highly accurate and reproducible measurements of the femoral sulcus from both the subchondral bone and the articular cartilage; measurement from the articular cartilage may be more relevant, because it constitutes the joint surface and is not possible to measure on radiographs.

Lateral trochlear inclination is the angle measured on the most superior axial image showing trochlear cartilage. It is the angle formed by the line drawn along the lateral trochlear facet and posterior condylar line. A lateral trochlear inclination angle less than 11° indicates trochlear dysplasia.[20]

Trochlear facet asymmetry and trochlear depth are both measured using the axial image 3 cm above the joint, and are both accurate measurements of trochlear dysplasia. Trochlear facet asymmetry is present if the medial trochlear facet length is less than 40% of the lateral facet length. Trochlear depth (deepest point of trochlear sulcus) is dysplastic if less than 3 mm at this same level (see **Fig. 12**).[20,21]

TIBIAL TUBERCLE TO TROCHLEAR GROOVE DISTANCE

The tibial tubercle to trochlear groove distance (TTTGD) has become the primary method for assessing excessive lateralization of the tibial tuberosity, a risk factor for patellar instability during flexion, sometimes referred to as excessive lateral friction syndrome.[20,21] This distance is measured on cross-sectional imaging using 2 separate but superimposed axial images, the first locating the tibial tubercle, and the second locating the deepest point/sulcus of the trochlea. The normal distance between 2 parallel lines that cross both of these points and are perpendicular to a third line tangent to the posterior aspects of both femoral condyles is defined as less than 15 mm, whereas greater than 20 mm is almost always associated with instability; measurement between 15 mm and 20 mm is considered indeterminate or borderline (**Fig. 13**).[20]

There are limitations in obtaining these measurements, because their accuracy and reproducibility are dependent on multiple technical factors. CT measurements in full extension were originally validated and are considered the gold standard, with recent efforts attempting to validate MRI measurements so they can replace CT.[33] Dedicated knee MRI coils have replaced both CT and MRI body coils for primary knee imaging. However, the knee rests in partial flexion within a dedicated knee coil, causing a mean

---

Fig. 12. Femoral trochlear dysplasia. (*A*) Lateral radiograph of the knee shows the crossing sign (*white arrowheads* showing decreased depth of the femoral trochlea with the floor of the trochlear groove crossing the anterior aspect of the lateral condyle), the double contour sign (*black arrowhead* showing anterior aspect of hypoplastic medial condyle) and a supratrochlear spur (*white arrow*), all findings associated with femoral trochlear dysplasia. Note also the near superimposition of the median ridge and lateral facet of the patella (*black arrows*), suggesting patellar tilt. (*B*) Lateral radiograph of the knee of another patient without femoral trochlear dysplasia for comparison shows normal trochlear depth (*white arrowheads*). Note also the lateral facet of the patella (*black arrowhead*) projecting anterior to the median ridge (*white arrow*), representing the normal relationship. (*C*) Axial radiographs of both knees show a shallow dysplastic femoral trochlea on the right. (*D*) Fat-suppressed proton-density-weighted transverse MRI of the knee shows dysplastic femoral trochlea with essentially no sulcus (*arrowheads*). Note loss of cartilage along medial patellar facet (*arrow*).

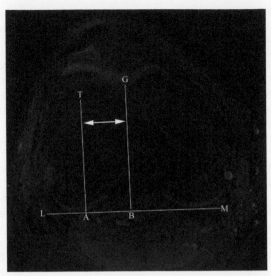

Fig. 13. Tibial tubercle to trochlear groove measurement. The image is digitally modified to show superimposed fat-suppressed proton-density-weighted transverse MRI through the knee at the level of the trochlear groove and at the level of the tibial tuberosity. A reference line, LM, tangent to the posterior aspects of the lateral and medial femoral condyles is drawn. The tibial tubercle to trochlear groove measurement is the distance (*double arrow*) between line TA (extending perpendicular from the reference line to the middle of the tibial tubercle) and line GB (extending perpendicular from the reference line to the deepest point of the trochlea). The distance in this patient was more than 2 cm, indicating excessive lateralization of the tibial tubercle.

TTTGD discrepancy of 8.6 mm. TTTGD measurements taken from knees scanned in dedicated knee coils may lead to patients being erroneously classified as normal.[34]

PATELLAR SLEEVE FRACTURE

Although pediatric patellar fractures are generally rare, patellar sleeve fractures are a common injury at the end of the patella seen only in skeletally immature individuals, comprising more than half of all patellar fractures in this demographic. Patellar sleeve fracture involves avulsion of a small osseous fragment along with a sleeve of periosteum and cartilage. These fractures are typically located at the distal pole, but may rarely occur at the proximal pole.[35] Although the small ossific fragment can be seen on radiographs, the cartilaginous fragment is not, and MRI is required to evaluate the full extent of the injury.[36]

PATELLAR FRACTURES

Patellar fractures may be caused by either direct trauma or indirect forces from the extensor mechanism. Indirect forces typically lead to transverse fractures, some with substantial displacement of the fracture fragments. By contrast, direct trauma more likely results in patellar fractures with comminution, articular injury, and anterior soft tissue damage. Vertical patellar fractures can occur but are rare. An axial view is helpful for evaluation but is difficult to obtain because of discomfort. A well-corticated fragment in the superolateral quadrant is more than likely part of a bipartite patella and not an acute fracture.[37]

PATELLAR DISLOCATION

Patellar transient lateral dislocation (PTLD) is an important but often challenging diagnosis. Although some cases are straightforward clinically, approximately half of all dislocations are not clinically suspected before imaging.[25] Patients are often unaware of previous dislocation and often deny such even when specifically asked; therefore, it is important to have high clinical suspicion when reviewing imaging.[38] Patellar dislocation usually requires predisposing factors of instability, including trochlear dysplasia, patella alta, and lateralization of the tibial tuberosity.[20] Acute patellar dislocations have a characteristic imaging pattern with high diagnostic accuracy, but chronic dislocations present a more challenging picture both clinically and by imaging.

Patellar dislocations are transient, nearly always relocated by the time of imaging, although abnormal lateral patellar tilt and subluxation often persist. The classic MRI finding that guides diagnosis is the bone contusion pattern. The acute osseous findings include a lateral femoral condyle contusion or osteochondral lesion, and a medial patellar facet contusion or osteochondral lesion; often the osteochondral fragment is attached to the medial retinaculum (**Fig. 14**). As many as 44% of patients have a concave impaction deformity of the inferomedial patella, a finding that is 100% specific for PTLD.[39]

The medial patellar restraints are commonly injured during lateral patellar dislocation; abnormalities are seen in 82% to 100 % of cases of previous patellar dislocation on MRI. Soft tissue injury patterns include injury of the medial retinaculum at its patellar attachment, midsubstance, or its femoral attachment. Tearing of the distal belly of the vastus medialis obliquus and injury of the MPFL at its femoral origin are likely the reason patients with acute patellar dislocation typically show tenderness along the adductor tubercle.[38] MRI findings of partial tears include intrasubstance or

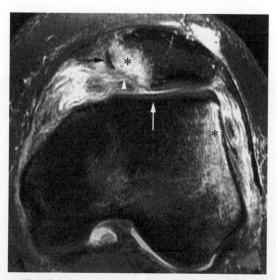

Fig. 14. Transient patellar dislocation. Fat-suppressed proton-density-weighted transverse MRI of the knee shows bone contusions in the medial aspect of the patella and the lateral aspect of the femur (*asterisks*), indicating recent transient patellar dislocation. Note also avulsed bone fragment from medial patella (*black arrow*), nonvisualization of disrupted patellar cartilage along medial facet (*white arrowhead*), and flattened femoral trochlea (*white arrow*), indicating dysplasia.

periligamentous edema, thickening, fiber irregularity, or partial discontinuity. Discontinuity with wavy or retracted fibers is characteristic of complete disruption, and joint fluid may extend through this defect.[40]

Joint effusions are typically present (although they may be absent in chronic habitual dislocations), containing layering fluid and blood (hemarthrosis); lipohemarthrosis contains an additional fatty component, diagnostic of fracture, which may otherwise be occult.[20] Chondral or osteochondral shearing injury is an important finding best depicted by MRI; it is crucial to examine the presence or absence of the underlying subchondral bone plate to distinguish these 2 injuries. It is also crucial to search for loose chondral or osteochondral fragments elsewhere in the joint (**Fig. 15**).[14]

Chronic findings related to patellar dislocation include ligamentous ossification within the medial patellar retinaculum at the site of injury.

TENDON ABNORMALITIES

Patellar tendinosis (PT) is one of the most common tendon abnormalities in athletes, particularly those involved in sports associated with repetitive jumping, such as basketball and volleyball. The chronic repetitive overload affects the patellar tendon typically at the inferior pole of the patella. In the acute phase, radiographs are likely to be normal. Chronic findings include calcification in the region of the patellar tendon or, rarely, intrasubstance calcification or ossification.[27]

On MRI, the normal patellar tendon is of uniform low signal intensity, has a convex anterior border, and is not thicker than 7 mm in anteroposterior diameter. MR features of PT include focal thickening of the proximal one-third of the tendon, a thickness greater than 7 mm, and focal T2 hyperintensity within the proximal tendon, most commonly involving the medial one-third of the tendon (**Fig. 16**). Other imaging findings include an indistinct posterior tendon border and edema in the adjacent Hoffa fat pad.[27]

Patellar tendon tears are infrequent and usually occur in adult men (<40 years of age) as a result of a high-velocity eccentric contraction of the quadriceps femoris, especially when a strong resistance in the flexed knee opposes it. Other predisposing

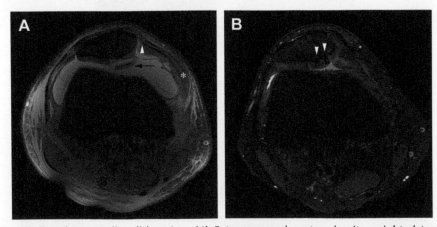

Fig. 15. Transient patellar dislocation. (*A*) Fat-suppressed proton-density-weighted transverse MRI of the knee in a patient with femoral trochlear dysplasia shows a large displaced cartilage fragment (*black arrow*) sustained after transient patellar dislocation. Note also tears of the MPFL (*white arrowhead*) and vastus medialis obliquus (*asterisk*). (*B*) Postoperative MRI of same patient shows fixation of cartilage fragment (*white arrowheads*).

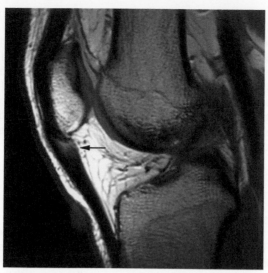

Fig. 16. PT. Proton-density-weighted sagittal MRI of the knee shows focal thickening and increased signal intensity within the proximal patellar tendon (*arrow*).

factors include chronic microtrauma and tendinopathy, previous tendon graft harvest for ACL repair, prolonged uses of steroids, and systemic diseases, such as chronic renal failure, diabetes, and rheumatoid arthritis.[41]

Radiographs in complete patellar tendon ruptures show patella alta, and an avulsion fragment may be present. MRI shows discontinuity of the patellar tendon, with increased T2 signal in the soft tissues from edema and hemorrhage (**Fig. 17**).[27]

Quadriceps tendon rupture (QTR) is a common extensor mechanism injury occurring most frequently in men in the sixth and seventh decades of life and is associated

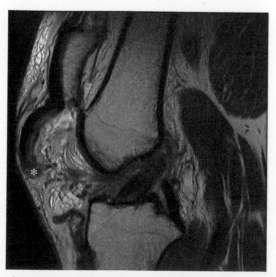

Fig. 17. Patellar tendon rupture. Proton-density-weighted sagittal MRI of the knee shows complete discontinuity of distal patellar tendon (*asterisk*).

with obesity, renal failure, and steroids. QTR may be partial, involving 1 or more layers of the quadriceps tendon, or complete (**Fig. 18**).[42]

Radiographs can show obliteration of the fat planes near the superior patella, suprapatellar soft tissue defect, joint effusion, patella baja, or an avulsed fragment arising from the superior patella. Diagnosis can be difficult in the case of partial rupture, and the superior specificity of MRI makes it the imaging modality of choice for accurately detecting rupture.[42]

On MRI, partial tendon tears are well evaluated on axial fluid-sensitive sequences. In cases of complete QTR, sagittal sequences are important to measure the distance between the torn edges, the quality of the underlying tendon, and the presence of hematoma.[27]

ANTERIOR BURSITIS

Prepatellar bursitis (PPB) or housemaid's knee is inflammation of the prepatellar bursa located between the patella and the subcutaneous tissue. With repetitive injury or microtrauma, the bursa becomes inflamed and a hemorrhagic bursitis can develop. In children, infectious PPB is common and the bursa is filled with pus. On MRI, PPB is diagnosed as fluid signal intensity in the prepatellar bursa distending it (**Fig. 19**). The bursa may be distended with simple fluid or hematoma. When large, the prepatellar bursa may extend and communicate with the superficial infrapatellar bursa or pretibial bursa.[27]

Infrapatellar bursitis (IPB), or clergyman's knee, involves the superficial infrapatellar bursa, which is located between the tibial tubercle and the overlying skin, as well as the deep infrapatellar bursa, located between the posterior aspect of the patellar tendon and the anterior aspect of the proximal tibia. On MRI, superficial IPB is diagnosed as a loculated collection anterior to the distal patellar tendon (see **Fig. 19**), and deep IPB manifests as a triangular fluid collection posterior to the inferior patellar tendon,[27] although a small amount of fluid is commonly encountered in the deep bursa normally.

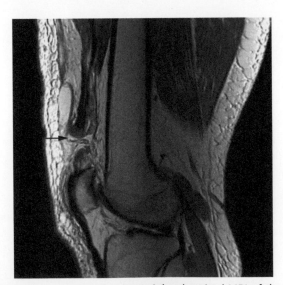

Fig. 18. Quadriceps rupture. Proton-density-weighted sagittal MRI of the knee shows complete discontinuity of distal quadriceps tendon (*arrow*).

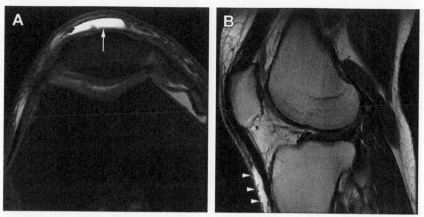

Fig. 19. Bursitis. (*A*) Fat-suppressed proton-density-weighted transverse MRI of the knee shows a fluid collection in the subcutaneous fat anterior to the patella, representing PPB (*arrow*). (*B*) Intermediate-weighted sagittal MRI of the knee shows a fluid collection in the subcutaneous fat anterior to the distal patellar tendon, representing superficial infrapatellar bursitis (*arrowheads*).

Morel-Lavallée Effusion

Prepatellar Morel-Lavallée effusions have recently been described in contact sports such as wrestling and football. The knee is an atypical location, because these lesions are classically encountered in other body parts, particularly the thigh and back. These effusions are caused by closed degloving shearing injuries at the junction of the hypodermis and muscular fascia (**Fig. 20**). The sheared hemolymphatic supply of the tissue then fills the perifascial plane with blood, lymph, and necrotic fat. In the acute to subacute setting, blood clot and debris may be found within an ovoid cavity of T2

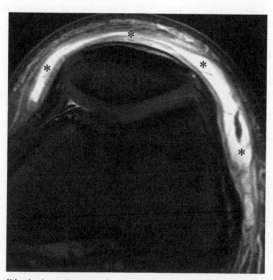

Fig. 20. Morel-Lavallée lesion. Proton-density-weighted transverse MRI of the knee shows an elongated collection of fluid anterior to the patella extending both medially and laterally (*asterisks*).

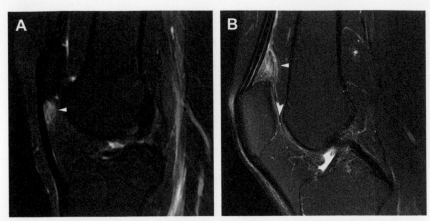

Fig. 21. Fat pad edema. (*A*) Fat-suppressed T2-weighted sagittal MRI of the knee shows edema (*arrowhead*) in the superolateral aspect of the Hoffa fat pad. (*B*) Fat-suppressed T2-weighted sagittal MRI of the knee shows edema in the suprapatellar (quadriceps) fat pad (*arrowhead*). Quadriceps fat pad edema is commonly seen and rarely causes clinical symptoms.

hyperintense fluid. As the hematoma becomes organized, the effusion may appear increased or intermediate in signal intensity on T1-weighted images.[43]

SUPEROLATERAL HOFFA FAT PAD EDEMA

Lateral patellar impingement is a clinical term used for AKP from patellar maltracking and impingement syndromes, and superolateral Hoffa fat pad edema is the most common correlative imaging finding by MRI, best seen on sagittal fat-saturated T2-weighted images (**Fig. 21**). Although there are many causes of abnormalities within various locations of the Hoffa fat pad, this superolateral location is not associated with prefemoral fat pad edema or quadriceps fat pad edema.[44]

QUADRICEPS FAT PAD EDEMA

Suprapatellar fat pad (quadriceps fat pad) edema with a mass effect on the suprapatellar joint recess is a common finding at MRI examinations of the knee and can rarely be a source of AKP. Best imaged on sagittal fat-saturated fluid-weighted sequences, the suprapatellar fat-pad is edematous with mass effect on the suprapatellar joint recess and, in some cases, it causes anterior scalloping of prefemoral fat pad (see **Fig. 21**).[45]

REFERENCES

1. Phillips J, Coetsee M. Incidence of non-traumatic anterior knee pain among 11-17-years-olds. S Afr J Sports Med 2007;19:60–4.
2. Kannus P, Aho H, Jarvinen M, et al. Computerized recording of visits to an outpatient sports clinic. Am J Sports Med 1987;15:79–85.
3. Kaufer H. Mechanical function of the patella. J Bone Joint Surg Am 1971;53: 1551–60.
4. Merchant AC, Mercer RL, Jacobsen RH, et al. Roentgenographic analysis of patellofemoral congruence. J Bone Joint Surg Am 1974;56:1391–6.

5. Laurin CA, Dussault R, Levesque HP. The tangential x-ray investigation of the patellofemoral joint: x-ray technique, diagnostic criteria and their interpretation. Clin Orthop Relat Res 1979;(144):16–26.
6. Hilfiker P, Zanetti M, Debatin JF, et al. Fast spin-echo inversion-recovery imaging versus fast T2-weighted spin-echo imaging in bone marrow abnormalities. Invest Radiol 1995;30:110–4.
7. Shindle MK, Foo LF, Kelly BT, et al. Magnetic resonance imaging of cartilage in the athlete: current techniques and spectrum of disease. J Bone Joint Surg Am 2006;88(Suppl 4):27–46.
8. Potter HG, Black BR, Chong le R. New techniques in articular cartilage imaging. Clin Sports Med 2009;28:77–94.
9. Tecklenburg K, Dejour D, Hoser C, et al. Bony and cartilaginous anatomy of the patellofemoral joint. Knee Surg Sports Traumatol Arthrosc 2006;14:235–40.
10. Wiberg G. Roentgenographs and anatomic studies on the femoropatellar joint: with special reference to chondromalacia patellae. Acta Orthopaedica 1941;12: 319–410.
11. Tyler P, Datir A, Saifuddin A. Magnetic resonance imaging of anatomical variations in the knee. Part 2: miscellaneous. Skeletal Radiol 2010;39:1175–86.
12. Kavanagh EC, Zoga A, Omar I, et al. MRI findings in bipartite patella. Skeletal Radiol 2007;36:209–14.
13. Link TM. MR imaging in osteoarthritis: hardware, coils, and sequences. Radiol Clin North Am 2009;47:617–32.
14. Endo Y, Stein BE, Potter HG. Radiologic assessment of patellofemoral pain in the athlete. Sports Health 2011;3:195–210.
15. Muhle C, Ahn JM, Trudell D, et al. Magnetic resonance imaging of the femoral trochlea: evaluation of anatomical landmarks and grading articular cartilage in cadaveric knees. Skeletal Radiol 2008;37:527–33.
16. Zeiss J, Saddemi SR, Ebraheim NA. MR imaging of the quadriceps tendon: normal layered configuration and its importance in cases of tendon rupture. AJR Am J Roentgenol 1992;159:1031–4.
17. Staeubli HU, Bollmann C, Kreutz R, et al. Quantification of intact quadriceps tendon, quadriceps tendon insertion, and suprapatellar fat pad: MR arthrography, anatomy, and cryosections in the sagittal plane. AJR Am J Roentgenol 1999;173:691–8.
18. Andrikoula S, Tokis A, Vasiliadis HS, et al. The extensor mechanism of the knee joint: an anatomical study. Knee Surg Sports Traumatol Arthrosc 2006;14: 214–20.
19. Warren LF, Marshall JL. The supporting structures and layers on the medial side of the knee: an anatomical analysis. J Bone Joint Surg Am 1979;61:56–62.
20. Diederichs G, Issever AS, Scheffler S. MR imaging of patellar instability: injury patterns and assessment of risk factors. Radiographics 2010;30:961–81.
21. Chhabra A, Subhawong TK, Carrino JA. A systematised MRI approach to evaluating the patellofemoral joint. Skeletal Radiol 2011;40:375–87.
22. Garcia-Valtuille R, Abascal F, Cerezal L, et al. Anatomy and MR imaging appearances of synovial plicae of the knee. Radiographics 2002;22:775–84.
23. Cothran RL, McGuire PM, Helms CA, et al. MR imaging of infrapatellar plica injury. AJR Am J Roentgenol 2003;180:1443–7.
24. Fenn S, Datir A, Saifuddin A. Synovial recesses of the knee: MR imaging review of anatomical and pathological features. Skeletal Radiol 2009;38:317–28.
25. Saggin PR, Saggin JI, Dejour D. Imaging in patellofemoral instability: an abnormality-based approach. Sports Med Arthrosc 2012;20:145–51.

26. Delgado-Martins H. A study of the position of the patella using computerised to-mography. J Bone Joint Surg Br 1979;61:443–4.
27. Samim M, Smitaman E, Lawrence D, et al. MRI of anterior knee pain. Skeletal Radiol 2014. [Epub ahead of print].
28. Phillips CL, Silver DA, Schranz PJ, et al. The measurement of patellar height: a review of the methods of imaging. J Bone Joint Surg Br 2010;92:1045–53.
29. Lee PP, Chalian M, Carrino JA, et al. Multimodality correlations of patellar height measurement on X-ray, CT, and MRI. Skeletal Radiol 2012;41:1309–14.
30. Shabshin N, Schweitzer ME, Morrison WB, et al. MRI criteria for patella alta and baja. Skeletal Radiol 2004;33:445–50.
31. Wissman RD, Ingalls J, Nepute J, et al. The trochlear cleft: the "black line" of the trochlear trough. Skeletal Radiol 2012;41(9):1121–6.
32. Dejour H, Walch G, Neyret P, et al. Dysplasia of the femoral trochlea. Rev Chir Orthop Reparatrice Appar Mot 1990;76:45–54 [in French].
33. Camp CL, Stuart MJ, Krych AJ, et al. CT and MRI measurements of tibial tubercle-trochlear groove distances are not equivalent in patients with patellar instability. Am J Sports Med 2013;41:1835–40.
34. Aarvold A, Pope A, Sakthivel VK, et al. MRI performed on dedicated knee coils is inaccurate for the measurement of tibial tubercle trochlear groove distance. Skeletal Radiol 2014;43:345–9.
35. Gettys FK, Morgan RJ, Fleischli JE. Superior pole sleeve fracture of the patella: a case report and review of the literature. Am J Sports Med 2010;38:2331–6.
36. Nath PI, Lattin GE Jr. Patellar sleeve fracture. Pediatr Radiol 2010;40(Suppl 1): S53.
37. Scolaro J, Bernstein J, Ahn J. Patellar fractures. Clin Orthop Relat Res 2011;469: 1213–5.
38. Schulz B, Brown M, Ahmad CS. Evaluation and imaging of patellofemoral joint disorders. Oper Tech Sports Med 2010;18:68–78.
39. Elias DA, White LM, Fithian DC. Acute lateral patellar dislocation at MR imaging: injury patterns of medial patellar soft-tissue restraints and osteochondral injuries of the inferomedial patella. Radiology 2002;225:736–43.
40. Earhart C, Patel DB, White EA, et al. Transient lateral patellar dislocation: review of imaging findings, patellofemoral anatomy, and treatment options. Emerg Radiol 2013;20:11–23.
41. Moretti L, Vicenti G, Abate A, et al. Patellar tendon rerupture in a footballer: our personal surgical technique and review of the literature. Injury 2014;45:452–6.
42. Perfitt JS, Petrie MJ, Blundell CM, et al. Acute quadriceps tendon rupture: a pragmatic approach to diagnostic imaging. Eur J Orthop Surg Traumatol 2013. [Epub ahead of print].
43. Borrero CG, Maxwell N, Kavanagh E. MRI findings of prepatellar Morel-Lavallee effusions. Skeletal Radiol 2008;37:451–5.
44. Subhawong TK, Eng J, Carrino JA, et al. Superolateral Hoffa's fat pad edema: association with patellofemoral maltracking and impingement. AJR Am J Roentgenol 2010;195:1367–73.
45. Tsavalas N, Karantanas AH. Suprapatellar fat-pad mass effect: MRI findings and correlation with anterior knee pain. AJR Am J Roentgenol 2013;200:W291–6.

Anterior Knee Pain in the Athlete

Laurie Anne Hiemstra, MD, PhD, FRCSC[a,b,]*, Sarah Kerslake[a,c],
Christopher Irving, MD[a]

KEYWORDS

- Anterior knee pain • Patellofemoral pain • Muscle strength • Quadriceps
- Patellofemoral kinematics

KEY POINTS

- Anterior knee pain has a multifactorial etiology.
- Routine clinical assessment of muscle strength in athletes may not detect deficits, so more challenging functional tests may be required.
- Nonoperative treatment is successful in most cases.
- Strong evidence supports treatment with multimodal physiotherapy.

INTRODUCTION

Anterior knee pain (AKP) is very common, affecting 1 in 4 athletes, 70% of whom are between 16 and 25 years old.[1,2] Considering that the patellofemoral joint is one of the most highly loaded joints in the human body,[3] the prevalence of AKP is not surprising. Athletes with AKP present a significant diagnostic and therapeutic challenge for the sport medicine caregiver. A clear understanding of the etiology of patellofemoral pain in this population is essential in guiding a focused history and physical examination, and achieving appropriate diagnosis and treatment.

The purpose of this clinical review is to provide an assessment framework and a guide for neuromuscular function testing, in addition to an overview of the causes and treatments of AKP in this challenging patient population.

SYMPTOMS

Patients with AKP complain of a variety of symptoms including pain, swelling, weakness, instability, mechanical symptoms, and functional impairment. Pain results from

Disclosures: Dr L.A. Hiemstra is a paid consultant for Conmed Linvatec. Banff Sport Medicine receives unrestricted research support from Conmed Linvatec, Centric Health, Genzyme.
[a] Banff Sport Medicine, PO Box 1300, Banff, Alberta T1L 1B3, Canada; [b] Department of Surgery, University of Calgary, 3330 Hospital Drive NW, Calgary, Alberta T2N 4N1, Canada; [c] Department of Physical Therapy, University of Alberta, 8205 114 Street, Edmonton, Alberta T6G 2G4, Canada
* Corresponding author. Banff Sport Medicine, PO Box 1300, Banff, Alberta T1L 1B3, Canada.
E-mail address: hiemstra@banffsportmed.ca

activities that load the patellofemoral joint, such as climbing up or down stairs, squatting, kneeling, and prolonged flexion of the knee joint.[4]

DIAGNOSTIC IMAGING

Diagnostic imaging including anteroposterior, true lateral, and skyline views should be obtained in all patients with refractory AKP. Computed tomography, magnetic resonance imaging (MRI), or ultrasonography should be considered when the history and physical examination determine that further imaging is required.

Table 1
Example clinical screening and advanced functional screening tests to assess neuromuscular control and strength in athletes presenting with AKP

Basic Strength and Muscle Length	Assessment	Example
Knee extensor strength	Assess in sitting with resistance at ankle and palpation of muscle tone. Can also be assessed as resisted straight leg raise in supine Monitor for lateral deviation of thigh, hip flexion, and/or trunk rotation due to muscle weakness or altered activation patterns[6]	
Hip abductor strength	Assess in side-lying with pelvis stabilized in mid-line and resistance above knee Monitor for hip and/or trunk flexion due to weakness or altered muscle activation patterns[7]	
Hip external rotation strength	Assess in supine with both the hip and knee flexed to 90°. Resist rotation at knee and ankle Monitor for hip flexion and/or poor through-range strength	
Quadriceps muscle flexibility	Assess in prone position with pelvis stabilized while examiner flexes knee. Compare heel with buttock distance Monitor for hip flexion, hip or thigh rotation to attain length[7]	

(continued on next page)

Table 1 (continued)			
Advanced Neuromuscular Lower Limb and Core Control	**Assessment**	**Correct Neuromuscular Control**	**Poor Neuromuscular Control**
Single-leg squat	Tests for core, gluteal, and quadriceps strength and control Assess depth of squat, dynamic valgus, side flexion of trunk, and pain[8]		
Hop down	Instruct patient to stand on one leg and then hop off step to land 10–15 cm in front of step Assess quality of movement, and evidence of dynamic valgus, hip drop, or rotation due to poor gluteal and/or core strength, lateral flexion of trunk, etc		
Balance	On BOSU ball or foam block, patient balances for up to 30 s Compare movement quality, range of motion outside base of support, dynamic valgus, hip drop or rotation, lateral trunk flexion, etc		
Active hip extension	Patient instructed to lift leg 5–10 cm off bed while lying prone. Palpate gluteal and hamstring muscle activation; ideally gluteals should fire first Assess for excessive motion, use of lumbar lordosis to achieve lift, altered timing of hamstrings and gluteal firing, and hip or trunk flexion		

Patients should be assessed bilaterally to compare limbs and monitor for any aggravation of symptoms.

TREATMENT PRINCIPLES

In all patients who present with AKP, a comprehensive knee, hip, and lower extremity evaluation including assessment of alignment, range of motion (ROM), lower limb and core strength, and functional movement patterns should be completed. Based on these findings, the combination of nonoperative therapy chosen should be selected using best clinical judgment. Nonoperative therapy includes relative rest, controlling inflammation, stimulating the healing response, and correcting biomechanics and neuromuscular control (**Table 1**).

Relative Rest and Activity Modification

Dye[5,6] challenged the way clinicians view the patellofemoral joint with his theory of the "envelope of function" to describe the pathophysiology of pain in patients with patellofemoral pain without overt abnormality. Dye portrays AKP as the loss of homeostasis of the tissues about the knee, with excessive mechanical overload exceeding the ability of the joint to repair itself in comparison with a homeostatic pain-free environment (**Fig. 1**). In an acute injury, relative rest will allow the tissue to heal and the symptoms will decrease. In more chronic cases, the physiologic responses to overload may cause daily activities to exceed the patient's pain threshold. This scenario represents a substantial therapeutic challenge, and requires significant patient education to rehabilitate the joint with pain-free loading.

The concept of the envelope of function includes 4 zones: disuse, homeostasis, overuse, and structural failure. Dye[5,6] proposed that all joints and musculoskeletal tissues respond to differential loading in one of these 4 zones. The outer limit of the homeostasis zone defines the envelope of function of the joint. The goal of treatment is to maximize the envelope of function as safely and predictably as possible.

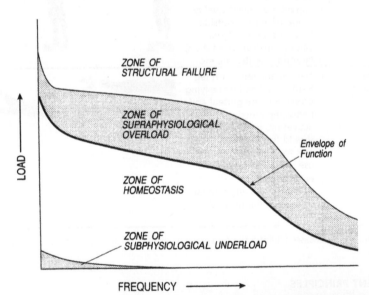

Fig. 1. The 4 different zones of loading across a joint. The area within the envelope of function is the zone of homeostasis. The region of loading greater than that within the envelope of function but insufficient to cause macrostructural damage is the zone of supraphysiologic overload. The region of loading great enough to cause macrostructural damage is the zone of structural failure. The region of decreased loading over time resulting in a loss of tissue homeostasis is the zone of subphysiologic underload. (*From* Dye SF. The pathophysiology of patellofemoral pain: a tissue homeostasis perspective. Clin Orthop Relat Res 2005;436:104; with permission.)

Methods to Control Inflammation

Cryotherapy

Ice packs and cold-therapy units are frequently recommended to athletes to reduce pain and inflammation secondary to AKP. Research has demonstrated the effectiveness of cryotherapy for reducing the internal temperature of the knee joint; however randomized controlled trials (RCTs) specific to AKP are lacking.[7,8] Park and Ty Hopkins[9] used an AKP model to demonstrate that cryotherapy produced a statistically significant reduction in pain. Cold therapy can also decrease the level of prostaglandins in the synovial tissue resulting in decreased inflammation,[10] reduce arthrogenic muscle inhibition caused by swelling,[11] and may facilitate vastus medialis motor neuron activity.[12] Cryotherapy may enable more effective quadriceps strengthening in patients with knee joint abnormality; therefore, despite the current lack of clear research evidence, cryotherapy is recommended as a mainstay of the conservative treatment of AKP.

Anti-inflammatories and analgesics

Medication treatments for AKP commonly include the use of analgesics such as aspirin or acetaminophen, and nonsteroidal anti-inflammatory drugs (NSAIDs). A Cochrane review of pharmacologic treatments for patellofemoral pain found no significant differences in clinical symptoms comparing aspirin with placebo, and limited evidence for the effectiveness of NSAIDs for short-term pain reduction.[13] Another Cochrane review assessing chronic musculoskeletal pain found that topical NSAIDs provided good pain relief, with no difference in efficacy between topical and oral NSAIDs.[14] The use of NSAIDs is controversial because of the absence of a histologic inflammatory response in several AKP abnormalities. There are also concerns that NSAIDs can interfere with the normal healing response of muscles and tendons. Short courses of NSAIDs may be considered when alternative approaches such as exercise, cryotherapy, analgesics, and other modalities have been unsuccessful, or when pain management is essential for participation in rehabilitation.

Methods to Stimulate Healing

Platelet-rich plasma

Platelet-rich plasma (PRP) is blood plasma, rich in platelets and associated bioactive factors, which can be delivered locally to an area that requires augmentation of the healing process.[15]

> "Even though the basic science data supporting the potential beneficial effects of growth factors in augmenting connective tissue healing are promising, the clinical benefits of using PRP to improve functional outcomes has not been universally realized."[15]

PRP injections have been studied for the treatment of tendinopathy and osteoarthritis. Filardo and colleagues[16] reported good medium-term results in the treatment of recalcitrant patellar tendinopathy with multiple PRP injections. The use of PRP has been rated by the American Academy of Orthopaedic Surgeons (AAOS) Clinical Practice Guidelines for the treatment of osteoarthritis of the knee.[17] Based on review of the literature, they were unable to recommend for or against the use of PRP for the treatment of knee osteoarthritis. The AAOS note that the quality of the literature was poor and that clinicians should use their best clinical judgment to make decisions.

Hyaluronic acid

Hyaluronic acid (HA) is a nonsulfated glycosaminoglycan distributed widely throughout connective tissue. Several meta-analyses have shown that HA injections can offer moderate improvement for symptoms of osteoarthritis of the knee. Although side effects have been reported with injections of HA, there is variability in the severity and incidence in the reports.[18–21] The use of HA has been rated by the AAOS Clinical Practice Guidelines for the treatment of knee osteoarthritis.[17] Based on a review of the literature, they were unable to recommend the use of HA for such treatment.

Other therapies

Acupuncture and dry needling have been proposed as effective treatments for AKP. Evidence from 2 RCTs demonstrated a statistically significant reduction in pain following acupuncture, lasting up to 6 months after treatment.[22,23] A few studies have indicated promising results from sclerotherapy and prolotherapy injections, although the lack of high-quality evidence prohibits definitive recommendation for use.[24] Sclerosing agents can be injected into areas of neovascularization, and prolotherapy is proposed to facilitate healing in conditions such as patellar tendinopathy. Systematic reviews and RCTs have demonstrated a lack of supportive evidence for the use of therapeutic ultrasound, iontophoresis, phonophoresis, low-level laser, transcutaneous electrical nerve stimulation, extracorporeal shock-wave therapy, biofeedback, and massage therapies. Recommendation for these treatments in patients with AKP should be based on the likelihood of benefit considering the duration of symptoms and the presenting symptoms.

Improving Lower Extremity Biomechanics

Patellar taping

Patellar taping has been shown to improve pain and function in patients with AKP when used in combination with strengthening exercises.[25–27] However, recent systematic reviews have drawn differing conclusions about the utility of taping for AKP. Warden and colleagues[28] concluded from their meta-analysis that a clinically significant reduction in chronic knee pain occurs with medially directed tape. Bolgla and Boling[29] stated that taping has minimal effect in treating long-term symptoms associated with AKP, but indicated that clinicians may consider patella taping as a short-term treatment to enable patients to perform pain-free exercise. Petersen and colleagues[30] also supported short-term use of a medially directed tape in combination with an exercise program. Callaghan and Selfe[31] determined in their Cochrane review that there was no statistically or clinically significant difference in Visual Analog Scale (VAS) pain scores comparing taping with no taping at the end of the treatment programs. Smith and colleagues[32] indicated that the research is controversial, and that tailoring treatment to the most suitable patients based on presenting characteristics may be the key to treatment success. A clinical trial by Lan and colleagues[33] investigating the response to patellar taping determined that it was an effective treatment for AKP, but was less effective in patients with a higher body mass index, larger lateral patellofemoral angle, and smaller Q-angle. Overall there is minimal evidence that taping significantly alters patellar alignment; however, it may increase the patellofemoral contact area leading to a decrease in pain, and thus enable relatively pain-free completion of exercise programs.[34–37]

Patellofemoral bracing

Similarly to taping, systematic reviews have reached differing conclusions about the outcomes of patellofemoral bracing. A meta-analysis assessing patellar bracing for chronic knee pain concluded there was disputable evidence from 3 low-quality studies regarding the efficacy of patellar bracing.[28] More recently, Swart and colleagues[38] concluded that knee braces offer no additional benefit over exercise therapy for pain and function in patients with AKP. Two reviews have noted the positive results of the Protonics bracing system in AKP, although further trials that examine the bracing system and exercise protocol separately are required.[29,38] Two reviews indicated that there is limited evidence to support the use of braces,[30,32] although Smith and colleagues[32] stated that it may be possible to use braces to reduce AKP onset in populations at risk. Bracing has also been shown in separate studies to decrease pain and improve function in patients with AKP.[39-41] Although the determinants of these positive results are not clear, they may be secondary to redistributed patella stress, enhanced proprioceptive input, and improved neuromuscular control.[29] Lun and colleagues[41] demonstrated that patellar bracing can improve the symptoms of AKP. However, these researchers also found that patellar bracing did not improve the symptoms of AKP more rapidly when added to a lower limb home-strengthening program. A recent quasi-experimental study demonstrated that patellofemoral bracing incorporating an infrapatellar strap significantly reduced pain and improved gait parameters in patients with AKP.[42] To definitively answer this clinical question the heterogeneity of trials, the variety of braces, and the quality of outcome assessment all require attention.

Foot orthotics
There is limited research regarding foot architecture and the use of foot orthotics as a treatment for AKP. It is also important that research has not consistently attributed foot pronation as a risk factor for AKP. Boling and colleagues[43] and Mølgaard and colleagues[44] determined that increased navicular drop was a risk factor for developing AKP; however, other studies have observed decreased foot pronation in association with AKP.[45] A clinical prediction rule, developed to identify patients with AKP most likely to benefit from foot orthoses, determined that individuals most suited to this treatment are older than 25 years, less than 165 cm in height, reporting their worst pain on a VAS at less than 53.3 mm, and with a difference in midfoot width from non–weight bearing to weight bearing of greater than 11 mm.[46] Barton and colleagues[47] demonstrated in an RCT that greater rearfoot eversion is a predictor of the benefit of foot orthotics in patients with AKP. A systematic review by Barton and colleagues[48] concluded that there is limited evidence for the use of prefabricated foot orthoses for short-term improvements in AKP. These investigators also reported that physiotherapy treatment combined with prefabricated foot orthoses is more beneficial than foot orthoses alone. Further well-designed studies focusing on assessment of gait kinematics and lower limb strength before and after interventions are needed to identify the cohort of patients with AKP most likely to benefit from foot orthotics.[29,30]

Stretching
Stretching of the quadriceps, gastrocnemius, and iliotibial band muscles have been investigated for AKP. In theory, tight hamstrings, gastrocnemius, or iliotibial band muscles could increase the patellofemoral joint reaction forces in full knee extension, whereas tight quadriceps could cause the same in full flexion.[49] A recent RCT demonstrated the benefit of quadriceps stretching for reducing pain in AKP, and recommended that this technique be included along with quadriceps strengthening in treatment protocols.[50] Studies investigating lower extremity stretching alone, or in combination with strengthening exercises or other physiotherapy interventions, have demonstrated improved AKP symptoms in up to 60% of patients.[51-55] Proprioceptive neuromuscular facilitation stretching techniques such as contract-relax may be more effective than traditional stretching programs.[56] Flexibility exercises and treatments are recommended as a component of the conservative treatment of AKP.

Strengthening

The effectiveness of exercise for reducing pain and increasing function in patients with AKP is widely supported.[29,30,32,57,58] A meta-analysis of RCTs determined that positive treatment results were evident with exercise interventions including knee extension, squats, stationary cycling, static quadriceps, active straight-leg raise, leg press, and step-up and -down exercises.[58] These investigators recommended a progressive program of daily exercises, including 2 to 4 sets of 10 or more repetitions over an intervention period of 6 weeks or longer. Two recent RCTs assessed the effectiveness of closed kinetic-chain exercises for AKP, and determined that these exercises can reduce pain and improve function.[59,60] Østerås and colleagues[60] also demonstrated that higher-intensity exercise over a 6-week treatment period resulted in statistically significant improvements 1 year after treatment in comparison with a low-intensity program.

A systematic review of conservative management of AKP from 2000 to 2010 concluded that both weight-bearing and non–weight-bearing quadriceps-strengthening exercises are effective for reducing pain in AKP.[29] This finding is consistent with those of the Cochrane review by Heintjes and colleagues[57] from 2003. In the more recent review, Bolgla and Boling[29] noted that although clinicians may prefer weight-bearing exercises to simulate functional activity, the use of non–weight-bearing exercise may be equally beneficial, particularly for patients with marked quadriceps weakness. A recent prospective study investigating weight-training for AKP demonstrated increased knee-muscle strength and patellofemoral joint contact area, potentially reducing mechanical stress in the joint and thereby improving pain and function.[61] One important factor highlighted in recent reviews is that exercises should be pain free.[29,32] The biomechanical stresses at the patellofemoral joint during exercise should be considered by prescribing clinicians, such as patellofemoral joint stress being lower from 90° to 45° of knee flexion during non–weight-bearing exercise, and also lower from 45° to 0° of knee flexion during weight-bearing exercise.[62]

Research protocols that include strengthening of the hip abductors and hip external rotators have reported significant decreases in pain.[29,53,63] A large RCT of military recruits found a 75% reduction in the incidence of AKP when hip exercises were included in training.[55] One study that included hip abductor, external rotator, extensor, and flexor exercises reported comparatively more significant improvements in pain, indicating the need for further study of total hip strengthening in AKP.[64] Bolgla and Boling[29] concluded in their recent systematic review that although hip exercises have been prescribed to obtain strengthening effects (ie, 3 sets of 10–15 repetitions), there is an indication that muscle endurance also needs to be addressed. These investigators stated that clinicians should consider exercise dosage focusing on higher repetitions (ie, 3 sets of 20–30 repetitions), in particular for AKP patients who participate in more demanding activities such as running and jumping.

The treatments available for AKP are numerous but lack evidence for their use, owing to insufficient research quality. The inability to recommend definitive therapeutic treatments for such a common disorder is disappointing, although it must be borne in mind that a lack of quality evidence for specific treatments is not proof that these treatments are ineffective. Each patient will present with unique symptoms and predisposing factors. With improving evidence, it will become increasingly more straightforward to tailor treatments unique to each athlete. Until such times, the authors encourage the use of best clinical judgment and application of available evidence-based medicine.

PATHOLOGY
Patellar Tracking

Abnormal patella tracking has been associated with disorders of the patellofemoral joint, including AKP.[61,65] In some cases deviation from normal tracking may be easily observed, but in other cases the differences may be subtle and therefore not recognized clinically. The patella translates medially in the initial 20° to 30° of knee flexion and then translates laterally[66]; however, there is no consensus regarding the normal amount of patellar tilt or rotation during this excursion.[67] Studies have demonstrated a more lateral patella position during initial flexion in AKP patients, but it is unclear if this deviation is present before the onset of symptoms.[68–70] Patella alta, patellar shape, and altered patellofemoral contact pressures are other potential risk factors for AKP.[69,71,72] Studies of quadriceps muscle function have demonstrated patella maltracking in combination with altered activation of the vastus lateralis (VL) and vastus medialis muscles.[73,74] Increased medial femoral rotation, rather than lateral patella rotation, has recently been demonstrated in AKP patients using weight-bearing MRI.[70] Abnormal patellofemoral alignment and tracking may be risk factors for AKP. However, further studies are needed to identify consistent changes in patellofemoral kinematics and whether these changes are a cause of, or a result of, patellofemoral pain.[65]

Soft-Tissue Pathology

Patellar tendinopathy

Patellar tendinopathy (jumper's knee) affects up to 40% of athletes involved in jumping sports such as volleyball and basketball, and appears to be more prevalent in men than women.[75,76] It can result in significant functional impairment in the athlete and can become chronic in nature, with one prospective study noting that patellar tendinopathy caused more than 50% of athletes to discontinue their sports career.[77] Tendinosis develops in response to chronic overloading of the tendon. Repetitive microtrauma interferes with the normal reparative process of the tendon.[78] Examination often demonstrates tenderness at the attachment of the patellar tendon to the distal pole of the patella. There is commonly palpable thickening of the tendon, and nodules may be palpated throughout the tendon. In less severe cases, functional testing such as squatting or hopping may be required to reproduce the athlete's pain. Ultrasonography may help confirm the diagnosis. There is evidence supporting eccentric strengthening as first-line treatment for patellar tendinopathy,[24,79,80] although systematic reviews have indicated the need for a multimodal approach to rehabilitation.[81,82] Injections have long been used for patellar tendinopathy. Corticosteroid injections may provide short-term benefit, but there is no evidence of long-term benefit and they are generally avoided because of the potential risk of patellar tendon rupture.[83] Studies on the use of PRP in this population demonstrate improvement in symptoms,[16,83] although significant side effects have recently been reported.[84] Studies of sclerotherapy and prolotherapy are currently not of sufficient quality to support definitive recommendation for their use. Surgical options include open, arthroscopic, and percutaneous techniques, and are generally reserved for recalcitrant cases nonresponsive to conservative management. In carefully selected patients surgery can be effective, although failure rates can from 20% to 30%.[85]

Bursitis

There are 11 bursae in the region of the knee joint, the most commonly affected being the prepatellar, infrapatellar, pes anserine, medial lateral collateral ligament, and semimembranosus.[86] In the athletic population common causes include overuse injuries and trauma, but can be associated with rheumatologic conditions, metabolic disorders, infection, and neoplasm. Symptoms and signs of bursitis include activity-dependent pain and focal tenderness over the affected bursa, often with associated swelling, stiffness, warmth, and erythema. Aspiration may be considered to rule out infection or to assess whether fluid analysis is required. Further imaging studies such as radiography, ultrasonography, and MRI may be considered as indicated. Treatment includes relative rest, activity modification, and protective padding over the affected bursa. Treatment to reduce inflammation, including intrabursal corticosteroid injections, may help. Surgery is not commonly required, but should be considered when appropriate nonoperative management has failed.

Pediatric patellar tendon abnormalities

Both attachments of the patellar tendon are subject to overuse or traction disorders in athletes with open growth plates. Osgood-Schlatter disease is a traction apophysitis of the tibial tubercle. The etiology is related to chronic loading of the patellar tendon–tibial tubercle junction, resulting in repeated minor avulsions with subsequent healing and repair attempts.[87] The disease usually occurs during the rapid phase of growth when the tibial tubercle is developing, with a similar prevalence in both genders, and bilateral symptoms are present in up to 30% of cases.[88,89] Sinding-Larsen-Johansson disease is an osteochondrosis of the inferior pole of the patella, and is another cause of AKP in the active adolescent population; it is more common in boys than in girls.[90] Symptoms of these 2 diseases usually include a gradual onset of activity-related pain localized to either the tibial tubercle or distal pole of the patella. Physical examination reveals tenderness and swelling or prominence at the site of injury, and in chronic cases bony irregularities may be palpable. Quadriceps and hamstring tightness are also common findings. Radiographs may be normal, or may show separation, fragmentation, and swelling of soft tissue at the site. Both conditions are usually self-limiting and respond to appropriate nonoperative management, including protective padding, activity modification, and methods to reduce inflammation, although it may take 12 to 24 months for symptoms to resolve.[91] Both long-term sequelae and surgical treatment are uncommon.

Iliotibial band syndrome

Iliotibial band syndrome (ITBS) is a common cause of lateral knee pain in athletes, especially in runners and cyclists, and in other sports such as rowing and swimming.[92–95] The literature surrounding the etiology, pathogenesis, and treatment of ITBS is controversial.[92,93] Current etiologic theories suggest that ITBS is associated with repetitive flexion and extension activities of the knee, in the setting of external and internal risk factors.[96–98] Activity-related pain in athletes is typically localized to the lateral femoral epicondyle (LFE) and/or lateral tibial tubercle.[95,96] Focal tenderness is common over the LFE, and associated swelling and crepitus may be present. Special tests include the Noble compression test to reproduce symptoms, the Ober test to evaluate iliotibial band (ITB) tightness, and the modified Thomas test to evaluate tightness of ITB, iliopsoas, and rectus femoris.[94–96] Treatment in the acute phase includes relative rest and avoidance of repetitive flexion and extension activities, methods to reduce inflammation, and addressing any muscle tightness and weakness.[95,96] A gradual and incremental return to activity is recommended after an athlete has become symptom free, with close monitoring for recurrence of symptoms.[95] Surgical intervention may be considered in cases refractory to conservative management, including arthroscopic debridement and percutaneous or open ITB release.[96]

Infrapatellar fat pad syndrome
Abnormalities related to the infrapatellar fat pad (IFP) can be a common but often over-looked cause of AKP in athletes. The IFP is an intracapsular but extrasynovial structure with rich vascular and nerve supply, and pain arising from IFP disorders can be signif-icant.[99] IFP syndrome may be caused by hemorrhage, inflammation, or impingement of the fat pad, and fibrosis may develop in chronic cases. Symptoms include anterior pain, often localized near the inferior pole of the patella, aggravated by forced exten-sion maneuvers and/or prolonged flexion. Physical examination may include tender-ness and fullness about the patellar tendon, and positive fat-pad impingement signs with forced passive hyperextension of knee and the Hoffa test.[78,100] In chronic cases findings may include catching and snapping, loss of extension, a palpably firm and enlarged fat pad, and decreased ROM of the patella. MRI can demonstrate hemor-rhage, inflammation, and fibrosis within the IFP.[101] Nonoperative treatment including corticosteroid or local anesthetic injections is often successful.[100] Surgical manage-ment includes arthroscopic resection of the IFP, which has been shown to be suc-cessful at relieving symptoms and restoring function.[102,103]

Plica syndrome
Plica syndrome can arise from 4 plicas within the knee: suprapatellar plica, infrapatellar plica, medial plica, and lateral plica. Plicas are present in approximately 20% of the adult population, and are normally asymptomatic.[104,105] Symptom development is most commonly associated with repetitive activity or direct trauma.[106] The medial plica is the most common symptomatic plica in the athlete.[107] When chronic, the plica can become fibrotic and inelastic, resulting in mechanical symptoms and erosive damage to underlying articular cartilage.[108] Typical symptoms may include AKP worsened by repetitive activity or prolonged sitting or standing, locking, catching, snapping, and giv-ing way. Physical examination demonstrates a tender, palpable thickened plica. The mediopatellar plica test has been described as a reliable test for diagnosing medial plica syndrome.[109] Nonoperative treatment has variable reports of success.[51] When indi-cated, arthroscopic resection has enabled successful long-term return to function.[110]

Cartilage Pathology

Chondromalacia patellae is a pathologic diagnosis describing degeneration of the cartilage on the undersurface of the patella.[111] It was originally described by Outer-bridge[112] in 1961 and then modified by the International Cartilage Research Society (ICRS). The ICRS classification is widely used in scientific literature as the reference standard. Chondral lesions of the patella comprise 11% of focal lesions found on arthroscopy.[113] Focal chondral lesions are usually diagnosed on MRI or arthroscopy, and these should initially be treated with activity modification, neuromuscular strengthening and stretching, injections, and other appropriate nonoperative manage-ment. In patients with ongoing pain after nonoperative management, arthroscopy is useful for characterization of the lesion, and may provide some therapeutic effect through debridement. More complex surgical treatment should include careful assessment of the underlying anatomy and biomechanics, such as malalignment and dysplasia. Surgical treatment directed at the lesion includes chondroplasty, microfracture, and chondral resurfacing techniques, such as osteochondral autograft or allograft and autologous chondrocyte implantation. Osteoarthritis of the patella, in contrast to a focal lesion, should be initially treated nonoperatively according to the AAOS Clinical Practice Guidelines.[17] Surgical management is limited, and may include arthroscopy, procedures to offload the patella such as anteromedialization (AMZ) of the tibial tubercle, and patellofemoral arthroplasty.

A subset of patellofemoral osteoarthritis is lateral hyperpressure syndrome, characterized by selective lateral patellofemoral compartment narrowing with patellar tilt. Patients present with pain and tenderness over the lateral patellofemoral joint. Skyline radiographs may show lateral narrowing of the patellofemoral joint space, patellar tilt, and lateral patellar osteophytes. MRI will identify selective lateral patellofemoral chondral damage. Standard nonoperative treatment includes lower extremity strengthening and stretching of lateral knee structures. Injections of HA or PRP may be of benefit in this population. Operative treatment includes correcting or improving biomechanical environment with procedures such as AMZ, lateral release for tilt, osteotomy to correct coronal malalignment, marrow stimulation techniques such as microfracture, and chondral resurfacing options.

Bone Pathology

Osteochondritis dissecans

Osteochondritis dissecans (OCD) is an acquired idiopathic disease of the subchondral bone that leads to death and subsequent collapse of the subchondral bone. The cartilage overlying the bone is unsupported and eventually fails, leading to separation of the cartilage and, eventually, loose body formation. Patients can present with pain at the site of the OCD lesion or with mechanical symptoms from a loose fragment. Diagnosis is generally made with plain radiographs, MRI, or bone scan. Treatment depends on the age of the patient and the stage of the lesion. Skeletally immature patients have excellent healing potential, and up to 66% have been shown to heal with nonoperative management including restricted activity, bracing, and limited weight bearing.[114] Poor prognostic factors include larger lesions, mechanical symptoms, patients approaching skeletal maturity, and MRI findings suggestive of instability.[115] Operative management for stable lesions includes retrograde or anterograde drilling.[116] For unstable lesions that are reducible, options include fixation with a compression screw or device, or osteochondral plug fixation.[117] A recent systematic review reported a 94.1% healing rate after surgical treatment of OCD lesions.[116] For lesions that require excision there is a variety of cartilage replacement techniques, such as osteochondral autograft or allograft, and autologous chondrocyte replacement.

Stress fractures

Stress fractures, though a less common cause of AKP in the athletic population, are worth mentioning. Approximately half of all lower extremity stress fractures are found in the tibia.[118] Stress fractures have also been described in the proximal fibula,[119] patella,[120] distal femur,[121] and tibial tuberosity.[122,123] Low-risk stress fractures include the posteromedial tibia, femoral diaphysis, and the first to fourth metatarsals.[124] High-risk fractures include the patella, femoral neck, anterior cortex of the tibia, medial malleolus, talus, navicular, fifth metatarsal, and the sesamoids.[125] Stress fractures occur when there is an imbalance between stress or breakdown of bone and the subsequent repair process. Stress fractures of the patella are most often transverse, and occur at the junction of the middle and distal one-third of the patella where the quadriceps tendon transitions into the patellar tendon.[119] Patients can present with a 2- to 3-week history of AKP-type symptoms or with catastrophic failure and a transverse fracture of the patella, with no history of significant trauma.[120] Intrinsic risk factors include menstrual history in women, metabolic conditions, level of fitness and muscle strength, alignment, and bone quality. Extrinsic risk factors include overtraining or a sudden increase in training, diet, and equipment.[126] Physical examination demonstrates tenderness over the site of the stress fracture. Radiographs are the initial imaging modality of choice, but may not show any evidence of stress fracture in the early stages. Radiographic features tend to lag behind clinical symptoms by several weeks. Bone scan and MRI are sufficiently sensitive to show the early changes associated with stress fracture.[127] Treatment includes identifying and modifying any contributing risk factors, and initial rest followed by a gradual, pain-free return to training, starting with nonimpact, followed by low-impact and then regular activities. Operative intervention is aimed at encouraging bone healing with stimulation at the fracture site with or without internal fixation. There is no definitive evidence for the use of other modalities such as bisphosphonates, growth factors, oxygen therapy, bone morphogenic protein, recombinant parathyroid hormone, ultrasound, or magnetic fields in the treatment of stress fractures.[128,129]

Trauma
Direct trauma to the patella occurs in several sports. It may increase intraosseous hyperpressure of the knee and may be an important factor in the etiology of patellofemoral pain.[130] The normal intraosseous pressure in the patella is between 10 and 20 mm Hg,[131,132] but this has been noted to increase to up to 70 mm Hg in conditions where stress is placed on the patella.[133,134] Patellar intraosseous pressure has been measured to be increased in patients with chondromalacia patellae in comparison with controls.[132,134] Raised intraosseous pressure can be the first step in a chain of events that eventually creates structural changes such as degeneration of articular cartilage. Increased intraosseous pressure may be a sign in all patients with patellofemoral pain, or may be an etiologic factor in patients with trauma or direct blow or bone bruise to the patella. However, further research is necessary in this area.

Bipartite patella
Bipartite patella occurs when one of the secondary ossification centers in the patella fails to close. This condition occurs in approximately 2% to 6% of individuals, and is often noted as an incidental finding on imaging. Males are affected more than females, with a ratio of 9:1, and 50% present bilaterally. Type III is the most common (75%), located on the superolateral pole of the patella.[135] Only 2% of bipartite patellae become symptomatic,[136] and often present as AKP after a trauma or direct blow to the patella. The diagnosis is made by plain radiography and palpable tenderness over the synchondrosis. Treatment is initially nonoperative and includes rest, activity modification, and quadriceps stretching. Operative management includes excision of the fragment with repair of the VL to the patella. Results are excellent, and allow a return to activity within 6 weeks.[137]

Patellar Instability

Patients with microinstability of the patella may present primarily with knee pain as the muscles attempt to stabilize the patellofemoral articulation, similar to as occurs in the shoulder where microinstability without gross dislocation can present as pain.[138] Patients can present with no injury history but may display predisposing anatomic factors such as generalized ligamentous laxity, high Q-angle, and valgus alignment.[139] Some patients will describe trauma ranging from mild to severe, but may not demonstrate the typical history of patellofemoral dislocation or ongoing instability. Patients may present with findings typical of patellofemoral instability, or signs of lateral laxity and apprehension may be subtle. Nonoperative treatment should initially include maximizing the neuromuscular function of the lower limb and core. Surgical management includes stabilization of the patella by medial patellofemoral ligament imbrication or reconstruction, in addition to addressing any predisposing anatomic risk factors such as alignment.

Neuromuscular Pathology

Quadriceps muscles

Muscle-strength deficits, diminished neuromuscular control, and altered muscle-firing patterns have been implicated as contributing factors to AKP.[32,140–143] Initially the research focus of AKP was on the quadriceps complex and, specifically, the evidence for a strength or timing imbalance between the VL and vastus medialis oblique (VMO) muscles. Lower peak torque knee extension has been confirmed as a characteristic finding in AKP patients, and has been demonstrated to be a risk factor for developing AKP.[143] One prospective study of chronic AKP patients with 7 years of follow-up determined that restoration of good quadriceps strength and function is essential for recovery.[144] There is also a trend toward a delayed onset of VMO relative to VL in AKP patients, although not all patients demonstrate this VMO-VL dysfunction.[143,145] Pattyn and colleagues[146] recently analyzed the factors that determine AKP outcome from a 7-week program of physical therapy, and determined that patients with a greater quadriceps muscle size, lower eccentric knee strength, and less pain have a better short-term functional outcome.

Hip muscles

Research has also examined hip-muscle weakness as a component of AKP.[147–150] Impaired gluteal muscle function is thought to lead to increased hip joint adduction and internal rotation during activities such as stair climbing, squatting, and sports.[147,148,151] Meira and Brumitt[150] concluded in their systematic review that there is a link between the strength and position of the hip and AKP, and that AKP patients present with a common deficit once symptomatic. A systematic review of hip electromyographic (EMG) studies presented moderate to strong evidence that gluteus medius muscle activity is delayed and of shorter duration during stair ascent and descent in individuals with AKP.[149] This study found some evidence that gluteus medius muscle activity is delayed and of shorter duration during running, and that gluteus maximus muscle activity is increased during stair descent. The investigators recommend that interventions focused on correcting these deficits, such as hip strengthening, biofeedback, or gait retraining, should be included in the treatment and research of AKP.

Muscle flexibility

Reduced lower extremity muscle flexibility has been cited as a characteristic of AKP patients, although study findings have been inconsistent.[141,152,153] Patients with AKP have demonstrated significantly less flexibility of the gastrocnemius, soleus, quadriceps, and/or hamstring muscles when compared with healthy control subjects.[152,154–156] Specific to athletes, a prospective study by Witvrouw and colleagues[155] discovered an association between tight quadriceps and the development of AKP, but not an association with tight hamstring muscles. Reduced iliopsoas and ITB length have also been demonstrated in some studies.[64,157,158]

Functional testing

Because routine clinical assessment of muscle strength in athletes may not detect deficits, more challenging functional tests may be more useful. Functional testing of athletes with AKP has demonstrated decreased performance on vertical jumping,[155] anteromedial lunge, step-down, single-leg press, and balance and reach tests.[153] However, research has not definitively concluded whether this lower functional strength capacity is a risk factor for, or result of, the disorder. A few sport-specific studies have demonstrated other muscle imbalances. An EMG study of trained cyclists showed altered muscle activation patterns in both the quadriceps and hamstring muscle groups in the athletes with AKP.[159] Runners with AKP demonstrate weaker or delayed activation of hip abductor muscles and an associated increase in hip adduction during running.[149,160–162] These results suggest that athletes with AKP are able to demonstrate distinct proximal neuromuscular control strategies.

Summary and recommendations

1. The findings of this clinical review demonstrate the multifactorial nature of AKP in athletes.

2. Most athletes with AKP can be managed nonsurgically.

3. A detailed history and thorough investigation of potential contributing pathology is essential to correctly tailor treatment.

4. Consider patellofemoral instability as a cause of AKP.

5. Perform a thorough lower limb assessment including screening for core strength and functional performance.

6. Ensure that relative rest and activity modification allow the knee to stay within the envelope of function.

7. Rehabilitation should focus on muscle strengthening, flexibility, and neuromuscular control of the core and lower extremity muscles.

8. Use best clinical judgment to select treatments that address the presenting anatomic and neuromuscular characteristics to optimally manage this condition.

9. Carefully progress rehabilitation and/or return to sport while monitoring symptoms.

10. Further high-quality studies are required to determine optimal treatments for AKP, including identification and matching of patient characteristics to effectively tailor care.

REFERENCES

1. DeHaven KE, Lintner DM. Athletic injuries: comparison by age, sport, and gender. Am J Sports Med 1986;14(3):218–24.
2. Devereaux MD, Lachmann SM. Patello-femoral arthralgia in athletes attending a sports injury clinic. Br J Sports Med 1984;18(1):18–21.
3. Dye SF. Functional anatomy and biomechanics of the patellofemoral joint. In: Scott W, editor. The knee. St Louis (MO): Mosby; 1994. p. 381–9.
4. Reilly DT, Martens M. Experimental analysis of the quadriceps muscle force and patello-femoral joint reaction force for various activities. Acta Orthop Scand 1972;43(2):126–37.
5. Dye SF. The knee as a biologic transmission with an envelope of function: a theory. Clin Orthop Relat Res 1996;(325):10–8.
6. Dye SF. The pathophysiology of patellofemoral pain: a tissue homeostasis perspective. Clin Orthop Relat Res 2005;(436):100–10.
7. Sanchez-Inchausti G, Vaquero-Martin J, Vidal-Fernandez C. Effect of arthroscopy and continuous cryotherapy on the intra-articular temperature of the knee. Arthroscopy 2005;21(5):552–6.
8. Warren TA, McCarty EC, Richardson AL, et al. Intra-articular knee temperature changes: ice versus cryotherapy device. Am J Sports Med 2004;32(2):441–5.
9. Park J, Ty Hopkins J. Immediate effects of acupuncture and cryotherapy on quadriceps motoneuron pool excitability: randomised trial using anterior knee infusion model. Acupunct Med 2012;30(3):195–202.

10. Stalman A, Berglund L, Dungnerc E, et al. Temperature-sensitive release of prostaglandin E(2) and diminished energy requirements in synovial tissue with postoperative cryotherapy: a prospective randomized study after knee arthroscopy. J Bone Joint Surg Am 2011;93(21):1961–8.

11. Rice D, McNair PJ, Dalbeth N. Effects of cryotherapy on arthrogenic muscle inhibition using an experimental model of knee swelling. Arthritis Rheum 2009; 61(1):78–83.

12. Hopkins J, Ingersoll CD, Edwards J, et al. Cryotherapy and transcutaneous electric neuromuscular stimulation decrease arthrogenic muscle inhibition of the vastus medialis after knee joint effusion. J Athl Train 2002;37(1):25–31.

13. Heintjes E, Berger MY, Bierma-Zeinstra SM, et al. Pharmacotherapy for patellofemoral pain syndrome. Cochrane Database Syst Rev 2004;(3):CD003470.

14. Derry S, Moore RA, Rabbie R. Topical NSAIDs for chronic musculoskeletal pain in adults. Cochrane Database Syst Rev 2012;(9):CD007400.

15. Arnoczky SP, Shebani-Rad S. The basic science of platelet-rich plasma (PRP): what clinicians need to know. Sports Med Arthrosc 2013;21(4):180–5.

16. Filardo G, Kon E, Di Matteo B, et al. Platelet-rich plasma for the treatment of patellar tendinopathy: clinical and imaging findings at medium-term follow-up. Int Orthop 2013;37(8):1583–9.

17. Brown GA. AAOS clinical practice guideline: treatment of osteoarthritis of the knee: evidence-based guideline, 2nd edition. J Am Acad Orthop Surg 2013; 21(9):577–9.

18. Rutjes AW, Juni P, da Costa BR, et al. Viscosupplementation for osteoarthritis of the knee: a systematic review and meta-analysis. Ann Intern Med 2012;157(3): 180–91.

19. Bannuru RR, Vaysbrot EE, Sullivan MC, et al. Relative efficacy of hyaluronic acid in comparison with NSAIDs for knee osteoarthritis: a systematic review and meta-analysis. Semin Arthritis Rheum 2013. http://dx.doi.org/10.1016/j.semarthrit. 2013.10.002.

20. Bellamy N, Campbell J, Robinson V, et al. Viscosupplementation for the treatment of osteoarthritis of the knee. Cochrane Database Syst Rev 2006;(2): CD005321.

21. Miller LE, Block JE. US-approved intra-articular hyaluronic acid injections are safe and effective in patients with knee osteoarthritis: systematic review and meta-analysis of randomized, saline-controlled trials. Clin Med Insights Arthritis Musculoskelet Disord 2013;6:57–63.

22. Jensen R, Gothesen O, Liseth K, et al. Acupuncture treatment of patellofemoral pain syndrome. J Altern Complement Med 1999;5(6):521–7.

23. Naslund J, Naslund UB, Odenbring S, et al. Sensory stimulation (acupuncture) for the treatment of idiopathic anterior knee pain. J Rehabil Med 2002;34(5): 231–8.

24. Gaida JE, Cook J. Treatment options for patellar tendinopathy: critical review. Curr Sports Med Rep 2011;10(5):255–70.

25. Osorio JA, Vairo GL, Rozea GD, et al. The effects of two therapeutic patellofemoral taping techniques on strength, endurance, and pain responses. Phys Ther Sport 2013;14(4):199–206.

26. Paoloni M, Fratocchi G, Mangone M, et al. Long-term efficacy of a short period of taping followed by an exercise program in a cohort of patients with patellofemoral pain syndrome. Clin Rheumatol 2012;31(3):535–9.

27. Crossley K, Cowan SM, Bennell KL, et al. Patellar taping: is clinical success supported by scientific evidence? Man Ther 2000;5(3):142–50.

28. Warden SJ, Hinman RS, Watson MA Jr, et al. Patellar taping and bracing for the treatment of chronic knee pain: a systematic review and meta-analysis. Arthritis Rheum 2008;59(1):73–83.
29. Bolgla LA, Boling MC. An update for the conservative management of patellofemoral pain syndrome: a systematic review of the literature from 2000 to 2010. Int J Sports Phys Ther 2011;6(2):112–25.
30. Petersen W, Ellermann A, Gosele-Koppenburg A, et al. Patellofemoral pain syndrome. Knee Surg Sports Traumatol Arthrosc 2013 [Epub ahead of print]. PMID: 24221245.
31. Callaghan MJ, Selfe J. Patellar taping for patellofemoral pain syndrome in adults. Cochrane Database Syst Rev 2012;(4):CD006717.
32. Smith TO, McNamara I, Donell ST. The contemporary management of anterior knee pain and patellofemoral instability. Knee 2013;20(Suppl 1):S3–15.
33. Lan TY, Lin WP, Jiang CC, et al. Immediate effect and predictors of effectiveness of taping for patellofemoral pain syndrome: a prospective cohort study. Am J Sports Med 2010;38(8):1626–30.
34. Malone T, Davies G, Walsh WM. Muscular control of the patella. Clin Sports Med 2002;21(3):349–62.
35. Christou EA. Patellar taping increases vastus medialis oblique activity in the presence of patellofemoral pain. J Electromyogr Kinesiol 2004;14(4):495–504.
36. Gigante A, Pasquinelli FM, Paladini P, et al. The effects of patellar taping on patellofemoral incongruence. A computed tomography study. Am J Sports Med 2001;29(1):88–92.
37. Derasari A, Brindle TJ, Alter KE, et al. McConnell taping shifts the patella inferiorly in patients with patellofemoral pain: a dynamic magnetic resonance imaging study. Phys Ther 2010;90(3):411–9.
38. Swart NM, van Linschoten R, Bierma-Zeinstra SM, et al. The additional effect of orthotic devices on exercise therapy for patients with patellofemoral pain syndrome: a systematic review. Br J Sports Med 2012;46(8):570–7.
39. Denton J, Willson JD, Ballantyne BT, et al. The addition of the Protonics brace system to a rehabilitation protocol to address patellofemoral joint syndrome. J Orthop Sports Phys Ther 2005;35(4):210–9.
40. Powers CM, Ward SR, Chan LD, et al. The effect of bracing on patella alignment and patellofemoral joint contact area. Med Sci Sports Exerc 2004;36(7):1226–32.
41. Lun VM, Wiley JP, Meeuwisse WH, et al. Effectiveness of patellar bracing for treatment of patellofemoral pain syndrome. Clin J Sport Med 2005;15(4):235–40.
42. Arazpour M, Notarki TT, Salimi A, et al. The effect of patellofemoral bracing on walking in individuals with patellofemoral pain syndrome. Prosthet Orthot Int 2013;37(6):465–70.
43. Boling MC, Padua DA, Marshall SW, et al. A prospective investigation of biomechanical risk factors for patellofemoral pain syndrome: the Joint Undertaking to Monitor and Prevent ACL Injury (JUMP-ACL) cohort. Am J Sports Med 2009;37(11):2108–16.
44. Mølgaard C, Rathleff MS, Simonsen O. Patellofemoral pain syndrome and its association with hip, ankle, and foot function in 16- to 18-year-old high school students: a single-blind case-control study. J Am Podiatr Med Assoc 2011;101(3):215–22.
45. Thijs Y, Van Tiggelen D, Roosen P, et al. A prospective study on gait-related intrinsic risk factors for patellofemoral pain. Clin J Sport Med 2007;17(6):437–45.

46. Vicenzino B, Collins N, Cleland J, et al. A clinical prediction rule for identifying patients with patellofemoral pain who are likely to benefit from foot orthoses: a preliminary determination. Br J Sports Med 2010;44(12):862–6.
47. Barton CJ, Menz HB, Levinger P, et al. Greater peak rearfoot eversion predicts foot orthoses efficacy in individuals with patellofemoral pain syndrome. Br J Sports Med 2011;45(9):697–701.
48. Barton CJ, Munteanu SE, Menz HB, et al. The efficacy of foot orthoses in the treatment of individuals with patellofemoral pain syndrome: a systematic review. Sports Med 2010;40(5):377–95.
49. Al-Hakim W, Jaiswal PK, Khan W, et al. The non-operative treatment of anterior knee pain. Open Orthop J 2012;6:320–6.
50. Mason M, Keays SL, Newcombe PA. The effect of taping, quadriceps strengthening and stretching prescribed separately or combined on patellofemoral pain. Physiother Res Int 2011;16(2):109–19.
51. Amatuzzi MM, Fazzi A, Varella MH. Pathologic synovial plica of the knee. Results of conservative treatment. Am J Sports Med 1990;18(5):466–9.
52. Crossley K, Bennell K, Green S, et al. A systematic review of physical interventions for patellofemoral pain syndrome. Clin J Sport Med 2001;11(2):103–10.
53. Fukuda TY, Melo WP, Zaffalon BM, et al. Hip posterolateral musculature strengthening in sedentary women with patellofemoral pain syndrome: a randomized controlled clinical trial with 1-year follow-up. J Orthop Sports Phys Ther 2012;42(10):823–30.
54. Rixe JA, Glick JE, Brady J, et al. A review of the management of patellofemoral pain syndrome. Phys Sportsmed 2013;41(3):19–28.
55. Coppack RJ, Etherington J, Wills AK. The effects of exercise for the prevention of overuse anterior knee pain: a randomized controlled trial. Am J Sports Med 2011;39(5):940–8.
56. Moyano FR, Valenza MC, Martin LM, et al. Effectiveness of different exercises and stretching physiotherapy on pain and movement in patellofemoral pain syndrome: a randomized controlled trial. Clin Rehabil 2013;27(5):409–17.
57. Heintjes E, Berger MY, Bierma-Zeinstra SM, et al. Exercise therapy for patellofemoral pain syndrome. Cochrane Database Syst Rev 2003;(4):CD003472.
58. Harvie D, O'Leary T, Kumar S. A systematic review of randomized controlled trials on exercise parameters in the treatment of patellofemoral pain: what works? J Multidiscip Healthc 2011;4:383–92.
59. Ismail MM, Gamaleldein MH, Hassa KA. Closed kinetic chain exercises with or without additional hip strengthening exercises in management of patellofemoral pain syndrome: a randomized controlled trial. Eur J Phys Rehabil Med 2013; 49(5):687–98.
60. Østerås B, Osteras H, Torsensen TA. Long-term effects of medical exercise therapy in patients with patellofemoral pain syndrome: results from a single-blinded randomized controlled trial with 12 months follow-up. Physiotherapy 2013;99(4): 311–6.
61. Chiu JK, Wong YM, Yung PS, et al. The effects of quadriceps strengthening on pain, function, and patellofemoral joint contact area in persons with patellofemoral pain. Am J Phys Med Rehabil 2012;91(2):98–106.
62. Steinkamp LA, Dillingham MF, Markel MD, et al. Biomechanical considerations in patellofemoral joint rehabilitation. Am J Sports Med 1993;21(3):438–44.
63. Earl JE, Hoch AZ. A proximal strengthening program improves pain, function, and biomechanics in women with patellofemoral pain syndrome. Am J Sports Med 2011;39(1):154–63.

64. Tyler TF, Nicholas SJ, Mullaney MJ, et al. The role of hip muscle function in the treatment of patellofemoral pain syndrome. Am J Sports Med 2006;34(4):630–6.

65. Song CY, Lin JJ, Jan MH, et al. The role of patellar alignment and tracking in vivo: the potential mechanism of patellofemoral pain syndrome. Phys Ther Sport 2011;12(3):140–7.

66. Amis AA, Senavongse W, Bull AM. Patellofemoral kinematics during knee flexion-extension: an in vitro study. J Orthop Res 2006;24(12):2201–11.

67. Katchburian MV, Bull AM, Shih YF, et al. Measurement of patellar tracking: assessment and analysis of the literature. Clin Orthop Relat Res 2003;412: 241–59.

68. MacIntyre NJ, Hill NA, Fellows RA, et al. Patellofemoral joint kinematics in individuals with and without patellofemoral pain syndrome. J Bone Joint Surg Am 2006;88(12):2596–605.

69. Salsich GB, Perman WH. Tibiofemoral and patellofemoral mechanics are altered at small knee flexion angles in people with patellofemoral pain. J Sci Med Sport 2013;16(1):13–7.

70. Souza RB, Draper CE, Fredericson M, et al. Femur rotation and patellofemoral joint kinematics: a weight-bearing magnetic resonance imaging analysis. J Orthop Sports Phys Ther 2010;40(5):277–85.

71. Connolly KD, Ronsky JL, Westover LM, et al. Differences in patellofemoral contact mechanics associated with patellofemoral pain syndrome. J Biomech 2009; 42(16):2802–7.

72. Luyckx T, Didden K, Vandenneucker H, et al. Is there a biomechanical explanation for anterior knee pain in patients with patella alta?: influence of patellar height on patellofemoral contact force, contact area and contact pressure. J Bone Joint Surg Br 2009;91(3):344–50.

73. Pal S, Draper CE, Fredericson M, et al. Patellar maltracking correlates with vastus medialis activation delay in patellofemoral pain patients. Am J Sports Med 2011;39(3):590–8.

74. Lin YF, Lin JJ, Jan MH, et al. Role of the vastus medialis obliquus in repositioning the patella: a dynamic computed tomography study. Am J Sports Med 2008; 36(4):741–6.

75. Lian OB, Engebretsen L, Bahr R. Prevalence of jumper's knee among elite athletes from different sports: a cross-sectional study. Am J Sports Med 2005;33(4): 561–7.

76. Zwerver J, Bredeweg SW, van den Akker-Scheek I. Prevalence of jumper's knee among nonelite athletes from different sports: a cross-sectional survey. Am J Sports Med 2011;39(9):1984–8.

77. Kettunen JA, Kvist M, Alanen E, et al. Long-term prognosis for jumper's knee in male athletes. A prospective follow-up study. Am J Sports Med 2002;30(5): 689–92.

78. DeLee J, Drez D, Miller MD. DeLee & Drez's orthopaedic sports medicine: principles and practice. 3rd edition. Philadelphia: Saunders/Elsevier; 2010.

79. Larsson ME, Kall I, Nilsson-Helander K. Treatment of patellar tendinopathy—a systematic review of randomized controlled trials. Knee Surg Sports Traumatol Arthrosc 2012;20(8):1632–46.

80. Jonsson P, Alfredson H. Superior results with eccentric compared to concentric quadriceps training in patients with jumper's knee: a prospective randomised study. Br J Sports Med 2005;39(11):847–50.

81. Malliaras P, Barton CJ, Reeves ND, et al. Achilles and patellar tendinopathy loading programmes: a systematic review comparing clinical outcomes and

identifying potential mechanisms for effectiveness. Sports Med 2013;43(4): 267–86.

82. Woodley BL, Newsham-West RJ, Baxter GD. Chronic tendinopathy: effectiveness of eccentric exercise. Br J Sports Med 2007;41(4):188–98 [discussion: 99].

83. Skjong CC, Meininger AK, Ho SS. Tendinopathy treatment: where is the evidence? Clin Sports Med 2012;31(2):329–50.

84. Bowman KF Jr, Muller B, Middleton K, et al. Progression of patellar tendinitis following treatment with platelet-rich plasma: case reports. Knee Surg Sports Traumatol Arthrosc 2013;21(9):2035–9.

85. Maffulli N, Longo UG, Denaro V. Novel approaches for the management of tendinopathy. J Bone Joint Surg Am 2010;92(15):2604–13.

86. Frontera WR, Silver JK, Rizzo TD. Essentials of physical medicine and rehabilitation: musculoskeletal disorders, pain, and rehabilitation. 2nd edition. Philadelphia: Saunders/Elsevier; 2008.

87. Ogden JA, Southwick WO. Osgood-Schlatter's disease and tibial tuberosity development. Clin Orthop Relat Res 1976;(116):180–9.

88. Kujala UM, Kvist M, Heinonen O. Osgood-Schlatter's disease in adolescent athletes. Retrospective study of incidence and duration. Am J Sports Med 1985;13(4):236–41.

89. Jarvinen M. Epidemiology of tendon injuries in sports. Clin Sports Med 1992; 11(3):493–504.

90. Medlar RC, Lyne ED. Sinding-Larsen-Johansson disease. Its etiology and natural history. J Bone Joint Surg Am 1978;60(8):1113–6.

91. Krause BL, Williams JP, Catterall A. Natural history of Osgood-Schlatter disease. J Pediatr Orthop 1990;10(1):65–8.

92. Falvey EC, Clark RA, Franklyn-Miller A, et al. Iliotibial band syndrome: an examination of the evidence behind a number of treatment options. Scand J Med Sci Sports 2010;20(4):580–7.

93. van der Worp MP, van der Horst N, de Wijer A, et al. Iliotibial band syndrome in runners: a systematic review. Sports Med 2012;42(11):969–92.

94. Lavine R. Iliotibial band friction syndrome. Curr Rev Musculoskelet Med 2010; 3(1–4):18–22.

95. Baker RL, Souza RB, Fredericson M. Iliotibial band syndrome: soft tissue and biomechanical factors in evaluation and treatment. PM R 2011;3(6):550–61.

96. Strauss EJ, Kim S, Calcei JG, et al. Iliotibial band syndrome: evaluation and management. J Am Acad Orthop Surg 2011;19(12):728–36.

97. Fairclough J, Hayashi K, Toumi H, et al. The functional anatomy of the iliotibial band during flexion and extension of the knee: implications for understanding iliotibial band syndrome. J Anat 2006;208(3):309–16.

98. Ellis R, Hing W, Reid D. Iliotibial band friction syndrome—a systematic review. Man Ther 2007;12(3):200–8.

99. Dye SF, Vaupel GL, Dye CC. Conscious neurosensory mapping of the internal structures of the human knee without intraarticular anesthesia. Am J Sports Med 1998;26(6):773–7.

100. Dragoo JL, Johnson C, McConnell J. Evaluation and treatment of disorders of the infrapatellar fat pad. Sports Med 2012;42(1):51–67.

101. Saddik D, McNally EG, Richardson M. MRI of Hoffa's fat pad. Skeletal Radiol 2004;33(8):433–44.

102. von Engelhardt LV, Tokmakidis E, Lahner M, et al. Hoffa's fat pad impingement treated arthroscopically: related findings on preoperative MRI in a case series of 62 patients. Arch Orthop Trauma Surg 2010;130(8):1041–51.

103. Kumar D, Alvand A, Beacon JP. Impingement of infrapatellar fat pad (Hoffa's disease): results of high-portal arthroscopic resection. Arthroscopy 2007; 23(11):1180–6.e1.
104. Duri ZA, Patel DV, Aichroth PM. The immature athlete. Clin Sports Med 2002; 21(3):461–82, ix.
105. Bellary SS, Lynch G, Housman B, et al. Medial plica syndrome: a review of the literature. Clin Anat 2012;25(4):423–8.
106. Lyu SR. Relationship of medial plica and medial femoral condyle during flexion. Clin Biomech (Bristol, Avon) 2007;22(9):1013–6.
107. Sznajderman T, Smorgick Y, Lindner D, et al. Medial plica syndrome. Isr Med Assoc J 2009;11(1):54–7.
108. Liu DS, Zhuang ZW, Lyu SR. Relationship between medial plica and medial femoral condyle—a three-dimensional dynamic finite element model. Clin Biomech (Bristol, Avon) 2013;28(9–10):1000–5.
109. Kim SJ, Lee DH, Kim TE. The relationship between the MPP test and arthroscopically found medial patellar plica pathology. Arthroscopy 2007;23(12): 1303–8.
110. Weckstrom M, Niva MH, Lamminen A, et al. Arthroscopic resection of medial plica of the knee in young adults. Knee 2010;17(2):103–7.
111. Grelsamer RP, Weinstein CH. Applied biomechanics of the patella. Clin Orthop Relat Res 2001;(389):9–14.
112. Outerbridge RE. The etiology of chondromalacia patellae. J Bone Joint Surg Br 1961;43B:752–7.
113. Hjelle K, Solheim E, Strand T, et al. Articular cartilage defects in 1,000 knee arthroscopies. Arthroscopy 2002;18(7):730–4.
114. Wall EJ, Vourazeris J, Myer GD, et al. The healing potential of stable juvenile osteochondritis dissecans knee lesions. J Bone Joint Surg Am 2008;90(12): 2655–64.
115. Pill SG, Ganley TJ, Milam RA, et al. Role of magnetic resonance imaging and clinical criteria in predicting successful nonoperative treatment of osteochondritis dissecans in children. J Pediatr Orthop 2003;23(1):102–8.
116. Abouassaly M, Peterson D, Salci L, et al. Surgical management of osteochondritis dissecans of the knee in the paediatric population: a systematic review addressing surgical techniques. Knee Surg Sports Traumatol Arthrosc 2013 [Epub ahead of print]. PMID: 23680989.
117. Miniaci A, Tytherleigh-Strong G. Fixation of unstable osteochondritis dissecans lesions of the knee using arthroscopic autogenous osteochondral grafting (mosaicplasty). Arthroscopy 2007;23(8):845–51.
118. Matheson GO, Clement DB, McKenzie DC, et al. Stress fractures in athletes. A study of 320 cases. Am J Sports Med 1987;15(1):46–58.
119. Drabicki RR, Greer WJ, DeMeo PJ. Stress fractures around the knee. Clin Sports Med 2006;25(1):105–15, ix.
120. Mason RW, Moore TE, Walker CW, et al. Patellar fatigue fractures. Skeletal Radiol 1996;25(4):329–32.
121. Milgrom C, Giladi M, Stein M, et al. Stress fractures in military recruits. A prospective study showing an unusually high incidence. J Bone Joint Surg Br 1985;67(5):732–5.
122. Tejwani SG, Motamedi AR. Stress fracture of the tibial tubercle in a collegiate volleyball player. Orthopedics 2004;27(2):219–22.
123. Levi JH, Coleman CR. Fracture of the tibial tubercle. Am J Sports Med 1976; 4(6):254–63.

124. Boden BP, Osbahr DC, Jimenez C. Low-risk stress fractures. Am J Sports Med 2001;29(1):100–11.
125. Boden BP, Osbahr DC. High-risk stress fractures: evaluation and treatment. J Am Acad Orthop Surg 2000;8(6):344–53.
126. Shindle MK, Endo Y, Warren RF, et al. Stress fractures about the tibia, foot, and ankle. J Am Acad Orthop Surg 2012;20(3):167–76.
127. Raasch WG, Hergan DJ. Treatment of stress fractures: the fundamentals. Clin Sports Med 2006;25(1):29–36, vii.
128. Carmont M, Mei-Dan O, Bennell KL. Stress fracture management: current classification and new healing modalities. Oper Tech Sports Med 2009;17(2): 81–9.
129. Young AJ, McAllister DR. Evaluation and treatment of tibial stress fractures. Clin Sports Med 2006;25(1):117–28, x.
130. Medscape General Medicine 1999;(1):1. Available at: http://www.medscape.com/viewarticle/717387.
131. Ficat RP, Philippe J, Hungerford DS. Chondromalacia patellae: a system of classification. Clin Orthop Relat Res 1979;144:55–62.
132. Bjorkstrom S, Goldie IF, Wetterqvist H. Intramedullary pressure of the patella in chondromalacia. Arch Orthop Trauma Surg 1980;97(2):81–5.
133. Arnoldi CC. Patellar pain. Acta Orthop Scand Suppl 1991;244:1–29.
134. Hejgaard N, Diemer H. Bone scan in the patellofemoral pain syndrome. Int Orthop 1987;11(1):29–33.
135. Saupe H. Primäre Krochenmark serelung der kniescheibe. Deutsche Z Chir 1943;258:386–92. http://dx.doi.org/10.1007/BF02793437.
136. Weaver JK. Bipartite patellae as a cause of disability in the athlete. Am J Sports Med 1977;5(4):137–43.
137. Weckstrom M, Parviainen M, Pihlajamaki HK. Excision of painful bipartite patella: good long-term outcome in young adults. Clin Orthop Relat Res 2008; 466(11):2848–55.
138. Ruotolo C, Nottage WM, Flatow EL, et al. Controversial topics in shoulder arthroscopy. Arthroscopy 2002;18(2 Suppl 1):65–75.
139. Hiemstra LA, Kerslake S, Lafave M, et al. Introduction of a classification system for patients with patellofemoral instability (WARPS and STAID). Knee Surg Sports Traumatol Arthrosc 2013 [Epub ahead of print]. PMID: 23536205.
140. Bolgla LA, Malone TR, Umberger BR, et al. Comparison of hip and knee strength and neuromuscular activity in subjects with and without patellofemoral pain syndrome. Int J Sports Phys Ther 2011;6(4):285–96.
141. Fredericson M, Yoon K. Physical examination and patellofemoral pain syndrome. Am J Phys Med Rehabil 2006;85(3):234–43.
142. Halabchi F, Mazaheri R, Seif-Barghi T. Patellofemoral pain syndrome and modifiable intrinsic risk factors; how to assess and address? Asian J Sports Med 2013; 4(2):85–100.
143. Lankhorst NE, Bierma-Zeinstra SM, van Middelkoop M. Factors associated with patellofemoral pain syndrome: a systematic review. Br J Sports Med 2013;47(4): 193–206.
144. Natri A, Kannus P, Jarvinen M. Which factors predict the long-term outcome in chronic patellofemoral pain syndrome? A 7-yr prospective follow-up study. Med Sci Sports Exerc 1998;30(11):1572–7.
145. Chester R, Smith TO, Sweeting D, et al. The relative timing of VMO and VL in the aetiology of anterior knee pain: a systematic review and meta-analysis. BMC Musculoskelet Disord 2008;9:64.

146. Pattyn E, Mahieu N, Selfe J, et al. What predicts functional outcome after treatment for patellofemoral pain? Med Sci Sports Exerc 2012;44(10):1827–33.
147. Prins MR, van der Wurff P. Females with patellofemoral pain syndrome have weak hip muscles: a systematic review. Aust J Physiother 2009;55(1):9–15.
148. Fukuda TY, Rossetto FM, Magalhaes E, et al. Short-term effects of hip abductors and lateral rotators strengthening in females with patellofemoral pain syndrome: a randomized controlled clinical trial. J Orthop Sports Phys Ther 2010;40(11): 736–42.
149. Barton CJ, Lack S, Malliaras P, et al. Gluteal muscle activity and patellofemoral pain syndrome: a systematic review. Br J Sports Med 2013;47(4):207–14.
150. Meira EP, Brumitt J. Influence of the hip on patients with patellofemoral pain syndrome: a systematic review. Sports Health 2011;3(5):455–65.
151. Powers CM. The influence of abnormal hip mechanics on knee injury: a biomechanical perspective. J Orthop Sports Phys Ther 2010;40(2):42–51.
152. Waryasz GR, McDermott AY. Patellofemoral pain syndrome (PFPS): a systematic review of anatomy and potential risk factors. Dyn Med 2008;7:9.
153. Loudon JK, Wiesner D, Goist-Foley HL, et al. Intrarater reliability of functional performance tests for subjects with patellofemoral pain syndrome. J Athl Train 2002;37(3):256–61.
154. Piva SR, Goodnite EA, Childs JD. Strength around the hip and flexibility of soft tissues in individuals with and without patellofemoral pain syndrome. J Orthop Sports Phys Ther 2005;35(12):793–801.
155. Witvrouw E, Lysens R, Bellemans J, et al. Intrinsic risk factors for the development of anterior knee pain in an athletic population. A two-year prospective study. Am J Sports Med 2000;28(4):480–9.
156. White LC, Dolphin P, Dixon J. Hamstring length in patellofemoral pain syndrome. Physiotherapy 2009;95(1):24–8.
157. Hudson Z, Darthuy E. Iliotibial band tightness and patellofemoral pain syndrome: a case-control study. Man Ther 2009;14(2):147–51.
158. Winslow J, Yoder E. Patellofemoral pain in female ballet dancers: correlation with iliotibial band tightness and tibial external rotation. J Orthop Sports Phys Ther 1995;22(1):18–21.
159. Dieter BP, McGowan CP, Stoll SK, et al. Muscle activation patterns and patellofemoral pain in cyclists. Med Sci Sports Exerc 2014;46(4):753–61.
160. Ferber R, Kendall KD, Farr L. Changes in knee biomechanics after a hip-abductor strengthening protocol for runners with patellofemoral pain syndrome. J Athl Train 2011;46(2):142–9.
161. Dierks TA, Manal KT, Hamill J, et al. Proximal and distal influences on hip and knee kinematics in runners with patellofemoral pain during a prolonged run. J Orthop Sports Phys Ther 2008;38(8):448–56.
162. Noehren B, Hamill J, Davis I. Prospective evidence for a hip etiology in patellofemoral pain. Med Sci Sports Exerc 2013;45(6):1120–4.

Patellar Instability

Jason L. Koh, MD[a,b,*], Cory Stewart, MD[b]

KEYWORDS

• Patella • Instability • Knee • Injury • Dislocation • Medial patellofemoral ligament

KEY POINTS

- Patellar instability is a common injury that can result in significant limitations of activity and long-term arthritis caused by recurrent injury.
- Recognition of the importance of bony alignment (tibial tubercle–trochlear groove distance), patella alta, trochlear dysplasia, and the femoral origin of the medial patellofemoral ligament (MPFL) is important.
- MPFL reconstruction requires precision in graft placement and minimal graft tension.
- Tibial tubercle osteotomy has a role in the treatment of bony malalignment and patellofemoral arthrosis.
- Trochleoplasty is a technically demanding procedure that involves potentially damage to articular cartilage and its role is still under investigation.

INTRODUCTION

Patellar instability is a common, debilitating injury that typically affects young active individuals,[1] and can result in significant limitations of activity[2,3] and long-term arthritis.[4] As such, patellar instability is a significant cause of morbidity in society. In the past, a variety of different treatments have been tried with varying degrees of success. There have recently been substantial advances in the understanding of the pathophysiology of patellar instability. Additional treatments and techniques have been developed as a result of this better understanding and these advances seem to provide superior results for the management of this disorder.[5]

Patellar dislocations account for approximately 3% of all knee injuries. The overall incidence is about 1 in 1000. Most patients who have patellar dislocations are young (aged 10–16 years) and female.[1,6] The rate of recurrence varies widely in patients treated nonoperatively, but, taken as a whole, first-time dislocators have a low rate of subsequent dislocation.[1,7] In patients who have had 2 dislocations, the risk of further injury is 50%.[1] In patients with known medial patellofemoral ligament (MPFL) injury confirmed on magnetic resonance imaging (MRI), the rates of redislocation are even higher.[8]

[a] Orthopaedic Surgery, NorthShore University HealthSystem, 2650 Ridge Avenue, Walgreen's 2505, Evanston, IL, USA; [b] Department of Orthopaedic Surgery and Rehabilitation Medicine, University of Chicago Medicine & Biological Sciences, 5841 S. Maryland Avenue, Rm. P207, MC 3079, Chicago, IL 60637, USA
* Corresponding author.
E-mail address: kohj1@hotmail.com

Clin Sports Med 33 (2014) 461–476
http://dx.doi.org/10.1016/j.csm.2014.03.011
0278-5919/14/$ – see front matter © 2014 Elsevier Inc. All rights reserved.
sportsmed.theclinics.com

Instability of the patellofemoral joint is multifactorial in cause. Abnormalities resulting in instability include the osseous structure of the patella and trochlea, the overall limb alignment, the integrity of the surrounding soft tissues, systemic conditions affecting connective tissues, and the patient's overall muscle tone.[9]

ANATOMY AND EVALUATION OF THE PATELLOFEMORAL JOINT
Anatomy

The patellofemoral joint comprises the undersurface of the patella and the cartilaginous anterior surface of the distal femur, the trochlear groove. The patella is a sesamoid bone embedded within the tendon of the quadriceps that has a complex gliding articulation with the femur. The patella serves to increase the mechanical advantage of the muscle for knee extension while protecting the knee.[10] The depth and steepness of the trochlear groove affects the inherent stability of the patellofemoral joint.[11,12]

At 2 months of gestation the patellofemoral articulation is in its adult form with normal knee mechanics and range of motion at birth. With maturation, the cartilage on the undersurface of the patella thickens to 6 to 7 mm, the thickest chondral surface in the body. The undersurface of the patella is composed of 2 unique facets: the lateral facet is longer and less steep to match the lateral aspect of the trochlea. Most patellar articulation with the trochlear occurs between the lateral facet of the patella and the lateral trochlear groove, with the medial facet only contacting the trochlear in deep knee flexion.[13]

Medial anatomic stabilizing structures include the patellofemoral (MPFL), patellomeniscal, and patellotibial ligaments, which are the main ligamentous structures that constrain lateral patellar motion. The strongest of these ligaments is the MPFL. The MPFL is a continuation of the deep retinacular surface of the vastus medialis obliquus (VMO).[14]

Cadaveric studies have shown that the MPFL with a tensile strength of 208 N contributes on average 50% to 60% of the total restraining force against lateral patellar displacement.[14] The MPFL has the greatest strain with the knee in full extension, and becomes lax as the patella enters the trochlea and the bony congruity of the joint provides most patella stability. The patella insertion of the MPFL lies between the superomedial and midmedial border of the patella.[14–17] Recent attention has been focused on the ideal femoral position to restore MPFL strain. The average width of the femoral attachment is 11 to 20 mm and the center of attachment is between the medial epicondyle and the adductor magnus insertion.[14,15,18,19] Several investigators have described this femoral attachment point with regard to radiographic landmarks.[20,21] This location, commonly known as the Schottle point, can be described as 1 mm anterior to the posterior cortex extension line, 2.5 mm distal to the posterior origin of the medial femoral condyle, and proximal to the level of the posterior point of the Blumensaat line.

The anatomy of the lateral soft tissue restraints is more complicated. The superficial layer consists posteriorly the superficial oblique retinaculum, and anterior lateral restraints largely consist of the expansion of the vastus lateralis.

The deep layer mirrors the medial structures and consists of the deep transverse retinaculum, epicondylopatellar ligament, and the patellotibial band, which attaches directly to the distal pole of the patella and sends fibers into the lateral meniscus and into the underlying tibia. The epicondylopatellar ligament does not attach directly to the tibia but attaches directly via the proximal and distal attachments of the iliotibial band (ITB).[22] As such, the tightness of the ITB influences the lateral stability force conferred by the lateral retinacular structures. The lateral retinaculum contributes approximately 22% of the soft tissue restraint to lateral translation, and is therefore an important stabilizer against lateral patella dislocation.[23,24] The medial and lateral retinacular structures are most effective within the range from 20° of flexion to full extension.[12,14,23]

Once the patella enters the confines of the trochlea, the bony anatomy allows for inherent stability of the patellofemoral joint. At 20° to 30° of flexion the patella is captured in the trochlea groove.[13] Because of this, symptomatic instability usually occurs before the patella is captured. Conditions resulting in patella alta are associated with an increased risk of recurrent patellar dislocations because the patella does not enter the trochlear grove until higher-than-normal levels of knee flexion are achieved. In addition, patients with patella alta have less surface area for articulation because the patella rides higher in the groove.[3,25,26]

Clinical History and Examination

Careful history taking and physical examination are important in the evaluation and treatment of patellar instability. Patient age and gender have relevance to recurrence risk. The number of previous clearly identified dislocation or subluxation events and the circumstances under which these occurred should be elicited. A history of general ligamentous laxity or dislocation in the patient or family should be obtained. Any previous surgery and the type of procedure(s) should also be recorded. Elements of the history that are relevant to the patient's functional status should be obtained, including types of physical activity engaged in by the patient during daily living, work, and sport; particularly those involving in cutting and pivoting. Identification of sensations of patella subluxation of dislocation should be differentiated from a feeling of giving way of the knee caused by reflex quadriceps inhibition. Pain location and activities that trigger it, particularly those involving loading of the patellofemoral joint, should be identified.

Physical examination of the patient with patellar instability should include an evaluation of overall limb alignment, including hip and knee rotation, and an assessment of generalized ligamentous laxity. Quadriceps muscle bulk, tone, and strength should be assessed, along with dynamic evaluation of limb alignment in single-leg squat maneuvers. The presence of apprehension with lateralization of the patella and the absence of a firm end point to lateral translation suggests previous dislocation and damage to the MPFL. Patella tracking (J sign), tilt, and mobility, as well as the presence of crepitus or effusion should be recorded. The Q angle in full extension may be falsely low in patients with medial side laxity,[9,27] so a knee-flexed Q angle may have greater reliability and more accurately identify the relationship of the trochlear groove to the tibia. The location of tenderness on the patella or along the MPFL should also be noted.

Imaging

Imaging of the patellofemoral joint can involve multiple modalities, including radiographs, bone scans, computed tomography (CT), and MRI. These different modalities can provide valuable information about the anatomy and also in some cases the cause of pain or instability for these patients.

Radiographs

A significant amount of information can be obtained by the use of carefully obtained radiographs regarding abnormal anatomy that can contribute to patellar instability, as well as information about arthritis and loose bodies. Standard anteroposterior and Rosenberg (posteroanterior 45° weight bearing) radiographs primarily provide information about the femorotibial joint and the presence of arthritis, but if carefully examined may also show loose bodies or small avulsion fractures from the medial patella. Lateral radiographs can provide a significant amount of information related to the patellofemoral joint.[28,29] When taken appropriately (with the condyles overlapping with <5 mm difference), lateral radiographs can provide extensive information not only regarding the presence of arthritis but also patella height, trochlear dysplasia, and patella tilt.

Patella height is typically measured using different ratios of patella size compared with tibial landmarks on a lateral radiograph (**Fig. 1**).[28] The Caton-Deschamps ratio compares the articular surface length of the patella and its distance with the anterior superior margin of the tibia. The Blackburne-Peel ratio compares the articular surface of the patella and its distance to a line projected forward on the tibial plateau. The Insall-Salvati ratio measures the overall patella length compared with the patella tendon. Normal values are in the 1:1 to 1.2 range, with values of 1:1.3 being considered definitely abnormal patella alta and possibly candidates for a tibial tubercle distalization procedure. The Caton-Deschamps and Blackburne-Peel ratios have been shown to have higher interobserver reliability than the Insall-Salvati ratio,[30–32] and also have the advantage of being able to show change when a tubercle osteotomy is performed. Therefore, one of these 2 ratios is preferred.

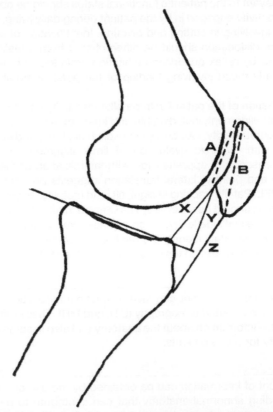

Fig. 1. Patella height ratios. All ratios 1:1 ± 0.2, Caton A/X, Blackburn-Peel A/Y, Insall-Salvati B/Z. (*From* Merchant AC. Patellofemoral imaging. Clin Orthop Relat Res 2001(389):17; with permission.)

Trochlear dysplasia can be identified on a perfect lateral radiograph by the presence of a crossing sign in which the trochlear groove line intersects the anterior femoral condyle rather than the anterior femoral cortex. The femoral condyles should overlap within 5 mm in order to assess the trochlea accurately. Dejour and colleagues[33] further classified the type of dysplasia by morphologic features of a supratrochlear spur (eperon sus-trochleen) and a double contour line (**Fig. 2**).[34]

Axial patellar views can provide information about loss of cartilage, spurs, and relative patella tilt and subluxation. The most commonly used in the United States is the Merchant view, taken at 30° to 45° of knee flexion. Multiple angles and indices have been described to measure the trochlea and patella relationship; however, up to 20% of normal knees have subluxation on axial views.[28] In addition, it is difficult to obtain more shallow angles of knee flexion. Because the patella is usually engaged in the trochlea by 30° the value of these views is limited for evaluation of patella instability. The relative importance of these measurements has diminished as improved axial imaging techniques have become available.

Bone Scan

Bone scans typically have less resolution than other imaging modalities, but can provide valuable functional information about metabolic activity of the bone. A diffuse uptake pattern is seen in patients with patellofemoral pain. A more localized pattern can be seen in patients with specific areas of overload or a symptomatic chondral defect causing increased activity in the underlying bone.[35] This pattern can guide treatment such as reducing activity or addressing focal chondral defects that contribute to pain.

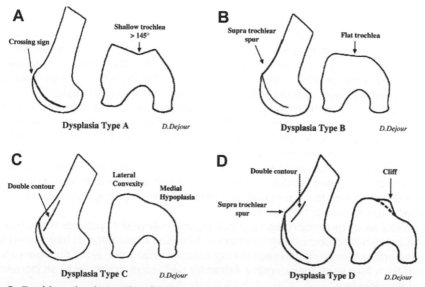

Fig. 2. Trochlear dysplasia. Classification of trochlear dysplasia. Type A: crossing sign, with trochlear morphology preserved (fairly shallow trochlea [>145]). Type B: crossing sign, supratrochlear spur, and flat or convex trochlea. Type C: crossing sign, with double contour. Type D: crossing sign, supratrochlear spur, double contour, asymmetry of trochlear facets, and vertical link between medial and lateral facets (cliff pattern). (*From* Dejour D, Le Coultre B. Osteotomies in patello-femoral instabilities. Sports Med Arthrosc 2007;15:40; with permission.)

CT Scan

CT can provide valuable axial imaging information at high resolution. The primary use has been to evaluate the anterior tibial tubercle–trochlear groove (TT-TG) distance. The mean value is 9 mm.[10] A TT-TG of 20 mm or more has a strong (>90%) association with patella instability.[33] CT imaging can also be used to evaluate relative femoral and tibial version, which can play a role in patella instability.

MRI

MRI has a valuable role in assessing articular cartilage and soft tissue injuries in patella instability. Articular cartilage damage on the medial patella facet and bone bruising of the lateral femoral condyle from relocation impact is common. MRI also has a valuable role in determining the location and extent of medial soft tissue injury that occurs with instability. In many cases, damage to the MPFL is evident. The location of damage to the MPFL injury can be variable, with injury occurring at the femoral origin (~50%), patella attachment (76%), and also midsubstance (20%); up to 49% have injury at multiple sites.[36] MRI has also been used to measure TT-TG distance using the articular cartilage of the trochlea as the center of the groove. However, MRI TT-TG measurements can underestimate the distance by a mean difference of 3.8 mm compared with CT.[37]

TREATMENT
Nonoperative Management

Decision making with regard to nonoperative treatment of patients with patellofemoral pain revolves around form and length of immobilization and timing and focus of physical therapy. In broad terms, the goals of early treatment of a patellar dislocation are to reduce swelling, strengthening the surrounding musculature, and improve knee range of motion.

Options for initial immobilization include casting, splinting, or bracing. Patients may either be casted in full extension or in partial flexion. In a long-term study of patients with primary patellar dislocations, those treated the most conservatively in casts for 6 weeks had the lowest risk of redislocation but the highest rates of stiffness. In contrast, patients treated with just a patellar brace had 3 times the risk of redislocation.[38]

Several investigators have compared early operative intervention with nonoperative management of first-time dislocators. A study by Buchner and colleagues[39] with 8-year follow-up of first-time dislocators found no significant difference between the surgically and conservatively treated groups with regard to redislocation, activity levels, functional outcomes, or subjective outcomes. A similar prospective, randomized study by Palmu and colleagues[40] compared 62 patients treated either operatively or conservatively and found no significant difference in subjective outcome, recurrent instability, function, or activity scores.

A smaller study by Arnbjornsson and colleagues[4] followed 21 patients with a history of bilateral patellar dislocations for a mean of 14 years. These patients had 1 lower extremity treated operatively, whereas the contralateral side was treated nonoperatively. In long-term follow-up, the operative extremity had worse arthritis and an increased risk of redislocation.[4]

Physical therapy for patients with patellar instability should center on closed-chain strengthening of the quadriceps and gluteal musculature, patellar taping, and proprioceptive exercises. Closed-chain exercises involving the gluteal musculature tend to increase the external rotation of the femur and as such decrease the Q angle during the gait cycle.[41] Strengthening of the quadriceps musculature, and in particular the

VMO, preferentially brings the patella medially in the trochlear groove. Patellar taping has been shown to control excessive patellar motion during therapy and serves to activate the VMO earlier than the vastus lateralis when climbing stairs.[42,43]

In deciding which first-time dislocators might be better served with early operative intervention, consideration must be given to the patient's degree of dysplasia and laxity. Patients who have dislocated more than once are likely to dislocate again and continued nonoperative management may not be indicated. As noted previously, patients with MRI-confirmed MPFL avulsion are also at high risk for reinjury[8] and early operative intervention should be considered.

Surgical Management

Indications for surgical management are related to patient pain and function. In many cases, patients have minimal symptoms at rest, but have significantly limited their functional activities because of apprehension.[44] Therefore, risk of recurrence is an important element for consideration in management. Other indications include a symptomatic loose body or cartilage lesions. In general, we have generally avoided surgery on patients who have experienced only 1 subluxation or dislocation event, because many of these patients do not have recurrent dislocation. A survey of National Football League team physicians indicates that most do not recommend immediate surgical management without a loose body.[9] However, if the patient has continued apprehension or a second dislocation event, we typically recommend surgery based on the high rate of recurrence. In addition, for those individuals with significant anatomic abnormalities, we consider early stabilization.

Surgical management of patella instability should be directed at correcting injured structures and, if the risk of recurrence is high, correcting significantly abnormal anatomic features that can contribute to increased risk, without resulting in excessive abnormal loads on the articular cartilage that can ultimately result in arthritis. This approach can include MPFL repair or reconstruction, tibial tubercle osteotomy with medialization and/or distalization, and in some cases trochleoplasty. Current surgical procedures are intended to recreate normal anatomy, rather than impose a nonanatomic constraint to motion. In general, the type and degree of abnormality dictates the particular techniques of surgical management used for an individual.

Arthroscopic and Minimally Invasive Techniques

Arthroscopic and minimally invasive techniques for the treatment of patellar instability include arthroscopic medial plication techniques and miniopen medial reefing techniques, and are typically limited to those patients with minimal amounts of bony malalignment or trochlear dysplasia, or as an adjunct to provide additional soft tissue balancing in patients who undergo bony procedures. The use of isolated arthroscopic lateral retinacular release is not supported by the literature and can result in increased lateral patella mobility[23] and even medial instability.[45] A survey of the International Patellofemoral Study Group resulted in a recommendation that isolated lateral release not be performed for patella instability.[46] For patients that require addressing medial retinacular laxity, we prefer the technique as described by Halbrecht,[47] in which a spinal needle is passed through the substance of the MPFL and a suture is passed through the lumen into the joint and retrieved through a cannula. The needle is then partially drawn back and then advanced the desired amount subcutaneously to pass again through the MPFL, where the suture loop is then retrieved and an arthroscopic knot is then tied intra-articularly. This procedure is repeated 4 to 6 times.

Published results of medial plication techniques have been satisfactory at short-term follow-up.[47–52] However, this technique in the presence of trochlear dysplasia has been shown to have a high early redislocation rate, and is therefore not recommended as an isolated technique in these patients.[53] It can help successfully reduce residual medial laxity in patients who have a tibial tubercle osteotomy.

Open MPFL repair of femoral side avulsions has also been described with reasonable results,[54–57] although a recent article from the Mayo Clinic described a 28% failure rate with this technique.[55] Specific technical aspects of this procedure are first to recognize that not all MPFL injuries occur at the femoral attachment, and, second, to clearly identify the femoral origin of the MPFL and verify that the strain behavior of the repaired tissue results in increased laxity of the tissue as the knee flexes. Repair at the femoral attachment if the damage is midsubstance or at the patella insertion does not satisfactorily address the underlying disorder. Nonanatomic or overconstraining repair is likely to either fail or result in excessive overload of the patellofemoral joint, and are to be avoided. We recommend careful identification of the general area of the femoral origin by radiographic imaging of the Schottle point, followed by an adequate incision to assess the anatomic landmarks of the adductor tubercle and medial epicondyle and the femoral origin of the MPFL, which lies in the saddle-shaped depression between them. The MPFL tissue can be brought to this point, and should show less tension as the patella engages the trochlea and the knee flexes. A suture anchor can be placed at the appropriate location and the ligament whip stitched to ensure that the tissue is firmly held. At best, this merely recreates the original, low-strength attachment of the MPFL.[58] We currently consider this in patients with minimal bony malalignment or dysplasia who have a clearly identifiable femoral avulsion of the MPFL, or as an adjunct to a distal realignment procedure in which residual medial soft tissue laxity can be related to a femoral avulsion.

MPFL Reconstruction

MPFL reconstruction is a technically demanding surgical procedure that is intended to rebuild the primary medial restraint to lateral patella translation. Various techniques have been described to replace the often atrophic or lax MPFL, typically with a graft that has significantly higher stiffness and ultimate load to failure than the native tissue. Grafts that have been used include free semitendinosus tendon or gracilis tendon autografts and allografts, bone-patella tendon-bone grafts, partial quadriceps tendon grafts, partial adductor magnus tendon grafts, and tibialis anterior allografts. Different techniques of attaching the graft to the patella have also been proposed, including looping the graft through tunnels in the patella, docking of the graft into a tunnel with an arthroscopic cortical button, anchoring the graft into tunnels with interference screws, attaching the graft to the patella using suture anchors, or suturing it to the retinaculum. Femoral attachment techniques include docking into a tunnel, suture anchors, or looping the graft around the adductor magnus tendon.[9,59–70]

Although a variety of different techniques have been proposed, it is critical that any reconstruction respects underlying biomechanical principles in order to be successful. Particularly with strong and stiff grafts, accurate placement and tensioning of the graft is important in order to provide the necessary constraint without limiting knee motion, overloading the medial patella articular cartilage, or causing medial patella subluxation. The normal strain behavior of the MPFL allows approximately 10 mm of lateral translation with the knee in full extension. The MPFL is under less strain after the patella is captured by the bony trochlea. Modeling of MPFL reconstructions has shown that as little as 5 mm of proximal malpositioning or 3 mm of shortening can lead to significant (>50%) increases in load on the medial patella facet.[71] Tension of 10 N can significantly increase patellofemoral contact pressures.[72] Abnormal placement can lead to significant complications such as patella fracture, loss of motion, or arthrosis.[73,74] However, nonanatomic placement of the MPFL is common,[75] with one recent article reporting that 64% of tunnels were malpositioned.[76] It is difficult to determine how many patients have abnormal tension applied to the graft, but a systematic review of the literature found a 26.1% reported complication rate and a 15.8% reoperation rate following MPFL reconstruction.[73]

Results of MPFL reconstruction show that, in most cases, good patella stability is achieved. Our recommended technique of MPFL reconstruction is used for patients with medial soft tissue laxity or atrophy and who have mild to moderate alignment abnormalities and dysplasia. A skin incision is created at superomedial to midmedial patella border, and dissection is carried through layer 1 to the medial border of the patella superficial to the synovial lining. Soft tissue is cleared from the superomedial corner to the midpatella in this area, and a bony trough is created using a burr. Suture anchors are then placed at the superomedial corner and midpatella.

The femoral insertion of the MPFL is initially identified using fluoroscopy to identify the Schottle point. A longitudinal skin incision is created that allows adequate dissection to clearly identify the adductor tubercle and medial epicondyle, and a guide pin is placed under a combination of fluoroscopic and anatomic guidance into the femoral insertion. The sutures from the suture anchor are then passed under layer 1 inferior to the VMO to the proposed femoral insertion of the MPFL. They are looped around the pin and set at an appropriate tension, and the strain behavior of the sutures is observed as the knee goes through a range of motion. If the femoral insertion site has been appropriately selected, the sutures should have decreased tension as the knee flexes.

Once the appropriate point has been selected, attention is again drawn to the patella. A semitendinosus graft is sutured into the prepared groove using the suture anchors. The free ends are brought under layer 1 to the guide pin, and again the strain behavior of the graft is evaluated through a range of motion. A tunnel of appropriate diameter is reamed over the pin, and the graft ends docked into the tunnel with the knee in 30° flexion and a spacer (such as a closed pair of Mayo scissors) can be used to avoid over tensioning. The graft is then secured with a soft tissue screw. The tension of the graft can be assessed as the knee goes through a range of motion; it should permit lateral motion at all points in early flexion, with approximately 1 cm of lateral motion with the knee in full extension.

TIBIAL TUBERCLE OSTEOTOMY

Tibial tubercle osteotomy has the advantage of being able to directly address some of the underlying biomechanical factors that predispose to patella instability in patients with an increased anterior TT-TG distance or with patella alta. In addition, an anteromedial transfer, as described by Fulkerson,[77] can unload damaged articular cartilage.[78,79] We typically recommend tibial tubercle transfer in patients with moderate to severe abnormalities of TT-TG, with patella alta with a Caton-Deschamps ratio greater than 1.4, or in patients with combined instability and distal lateral articular cartilage lesions. Various types of tibial tubercle osteotomies have been proposed; the most commonly used are the Elmslie-Trillat medial transfer[80] and the Fulkerson-type anteromedialization tibial tubercle transfer. The Fulkerson anteromedialization has the advantage of being able to unload the distal and lateral articular cartilage of the patella as well as improve patella tracking. The amount of distal unloading can be increased by increasing the obliquity of the osteotomy. The Hauser procedure, which consists of a posteromedial transfer of tubercle, has a high failure rate as well as an increased rate of arthrosis from the increased forces across the joint, and is not recommended.

Complications associated with tibial tubercle osteotomy include overmedialization, which can be avoided with appropriate preoperative planning of the distance the patella is transferred; tubercle nonunion; tubercle fracture; and tibia fracture.[81] Tubercle nonunion is uncommon and is typically related to inadequate fixation and a poor host environment. Tubercle fracture can be avoided by creating a shingle of appropriate length and width; typically, a minimum of 5 cm length is suggested. Tibia fracture is a greater risk with deeper, more oblique cuts,[81] and has occurred in the presence of accelerated weight-bearing protocols. Therefore, protected weight bearing for 6 to 8 weeks is recommended.[82,83]

Our technique has been previously described.[84] In brief, following a careful arthroscopic evaluation of the joint, a longitudinal incision 5 cm long is made at the tibial tubercle. The medial and lateral borders of the tubercle are defined and the anterolateral musculature is carefully elevated from the tibia. A 5 cm long oblique, tapered osteotomy is made using an oscillating saw cooled with regular saline irrigation angling the blade from anteromedial to lateral. The proximal portion of the osteotomy is completed manually using osteotomes. The tubercle is medialized approximately 1 cm, and provisionally fixed with a Kirschner wire. If necessary, the shingle is mobilized at the tip and shifted distally to correct for concomitant patella alta. Patella tracking and stability are then assessed clinically and arthroscopically; if adequate, without over medialization, the shingle is secured with bicortical compression lag screw fixation to the posterior tibial cortex. Care is taken to drill with the knee flexed 90° to allow posterior neurovascular structures to fall away from the posterior tibia and avoid plunging the drill bit. Patella tracking is then reassessed. If there is residual lateral laxity, then medial repair or imbrication are performed until good patella balance is achieved. It is unusual to require formal MPFL reconstruction when there has been a tibial tubercle transfer; however, if patients are able to dislocate with the knee flexed, a combined MPFL reconstruction along with a tubercle osteotomy may be necessary.

Results after tibial tubercle transfer for instability are generally good; however, recurrent instability and pain can still occur. At longer term follow-up (>5 years) 80% of patients reported good to excellent outcomes.[85] Results seem to be worse in patients with articular cartilage damage.

Trochleoplasty

Trochleoplasty has been considered by several investigators for the treatment of severe trochlear dysplasia in patients with instability. Several types of trochleoplasty have been described, including lateral elevation (Albee)–type trochleoplasty,[86] a deepening trochleoplasty as described by Dejour,[87] and a resection trochleoplasty (Goutallier)[88] in which the proximal bump is flattened to the femoral cortex without deepening of the groove. Peterson Vasiliadis[89] has also described a proximal trochleoplasty, which is primarily creation of a proximal groove extending into the dysplastic trochlea. The Albee lateral elevation osteotomy can lead to increased patellofemoral contact pressures. The deepening trochleoplasty requires the elevation of an osteochondral flake of bone, followed by resection to create an underlying groove and compression of the osteochondral piece into the new groove. This technique has the risk of articular cartilage damage, although biopsy specimens show preservation of normal hyaline cartilage architecture. Both the elevation and deepening trochleoplasties run the risk of incongruity with respect to the patella. The resection trochleoplasty has less risk of articular cartilage damage but also confers less stability.[86]

This operation is technically challenging and has a significant risk of complications, including arthrofibrosis and arthritis.[86,90,91] In most of these procedures an intra-articular fracture is created at the patellofemoral joint. Blond and Schottle[92] described an arthroscopic trochleoplasty technique that is demanding to perform, with good results, and improved surgical instrumentation may allow a more reproducible technique.

SUMMARY

Patella instability can cause significant pain and functional limitations. Several factors can predispose to patella instability, such as ligamentous laxity, increased anterior TT-TG distance, patella alta, and trochlear dysplasia. Acquired factors include MPFL injury or abnormal quadriceps function. In many cases, first-time dislocation can successfully be managed with physical therapy and other nonoperative management; however, more than one dislocation significantly increases the chance of recurrence. Surgical management can improve stability, but should be tailored to the injuries and anatomic risk factors for recurrent dislocation. Isolated lateral release is not supported by current literature and increases the risk of iatrogenic medial instability. Medial repair is usually reserved for patients with largely normal anatomy. MPFL reconstruction can successfully stabilize patients with medial soft tissue injury but is a technically demanding procedure with a high complication rate and risks of pain and arthrosis. Tibial tubercle osteotomy can address bony malalignment and also unload certain articular cartilage lesions while improving stability. Trochleoplasty may be indicated in individuals with a severely dysplastic trochlea that cannot otherwise be stabilized. A combination of procedures may be necessary to fully address the multiple factors involved in causing pain, loss of function, and risk of recurrence in patients with patellar instability.

REFERENCES

1. Fithian DC, Paxton EW, Stone ML, et al. Epidemiology and natural history of acute patellar dislocation. Am J Sports Med 2004;32(5):1114–21.
2. Hawkins RJ, Bell RH, Anisette G. Acute patellar dislocations. The natural history. Am J Sports Med 1986;14(2):117–20.
3. Atkin DM, Fithian DC, Marangi KS, et al. Characteristics of patients with primary acute lateral patellar dislocation and their recovery within the first 6 months of injury. Am J Sports Med 2000;28(4):472–9.
4. Arnbjornsson A, Egund N, Rydling O, et al. The natural history of recurrent dislocation of the patella. Long-term results of conservative and operative treatment. J Bone Joint Surg Br 1992;74(1):140–2.
5. White BJ, Sherman OH. Patellofemoral instability. Bull NYU Hosp Jt Dis 2009; 67(1):22–9.
6. Hsiao M, Owens BD, Burks R, et al. Incidence of acute traumatic patellar dislocation among active-duty United States military service members. Am J Sports Med 2010;38(10):1997–2004.
7. Hing CB, Smith TO, Donell S, et al. Surgical versus non-surgical interventions for treating patellar dislocation. Cochrane Database Syst Rev 2011;(11):CD008106.
8. Sillanpaa PJ, Peltola E, Mattila VM, et al. Femoral avulsion of the medial patellofemoral ligament after primary traumatic patellar dislocation predicts subsequent instability in men: a mean 7-year nonoperative follow-up study. Am J Sports Med 2009;37(8):1513–21.
9. Colvin AC, West RV. Patellar instability. J Bone Joint Surg Am 2008;90(12): 2751–62.
10. Rhee SJ, Pavlou G, Oakley J, et al. Modern management of patellar instability. Int Orthop 2012;36(12):2447–56.

11. Amis AA, Oguz C, Bull AM, et al. The effect of trochleoplasty on patellar stability and kinematics: a biomechanical study in vitro. J Bone Joint Surg Br 2008;90(7): 864–9.
12. Senavongse W, Amis AA. The effects of articular, retinacular, or muscular deficiencies on patellofemoral joint stability: a biomechanical study in vitro. J Bone Joint Surg Br 2005;87(4):577–82.
13. Amis AA, Senavongse W, Bull AM. Patellofemoral kinematics during knee flexion-extension: an in vitro study. J Orthop Res 2006;24(12):2201–11.
14. Amis AA, Firer P, Mountney J, et al. Anatomy and biomechanics of the medial patellofemoral ligament. Knee 2003;10(3):215–20.
15. Baldwin JL. The anatomy of the medial patellofemoral ligament. Am J Sports Med 2009;37(12):2355–61.
16. Philippot R, Chouteau J, Wegrzyn J, et al. Medial patellofemoral ligament anatomy: implications for its surgical reconstruction. Knee Surg Sports Traumatol Arthrosc 2009;17(5):475–9.
17. Steensen RN, Dopirak RM, McDonald WG 3rd. The anatomy and isometry of the medial patellofemoral ligament: implications for reconstruction. Am J Sports Med 2004;32(6):1509–13.
18. Mochizuki T, Nimura A, Tateishi T, et al. Anatomic study of the attachment of the medial patellofemoral ligament and its characteristic relationships to the vastus intermedius. Knee Surg Sports Traumatol Arthrosc 2013;21(2):305–10.
19. LaPrade RF, Engebretsen AH, Ly TV, et al. The anatomy of the medial part of the knee. J Bone Joint Surg Am 2007;89(9):2000–10.
20. Schottle PB, Schmeling A, Rosenstiel N, et al. Radiographic landmarks for femoral tunnel placement in medial patellofemoral ligament reconstruction. Am J Sports Med 2007;35(5):801–4.
21. Redfern J, Kamath G, Burks R. Anatomical confirmation of the use of radiographic landmarks in medial patellofemoral ligament reconstruction. Am J Sports Med 2010;38(2):293–7.
22. Fulkerson JP, Gossling HR. Anatomy of the knee joint lateral retinaculum. Clin Orthop Relat Res 1980;(153):183–8.
23. Christoforakis J, Bull AM, Strachan RK, et al. Effects of lateral retinacular release on the lateral stability of the patella. Knee Surg Sports Traumatol Arthrosc 2006; 14(3):273–7.
24. Feller JA, Amis AA, Andrish JT, et al. Surgical biomechanics of the patellofemoral joint. Arthroscopy 2007;23(5):542–53.
25. Geenen E, Molenaers G, Martens M. Patella alta in patellofemoral instability. Acta Orthop Belg 1989;55(3):387–93.
26. Insall J, Goldberg V, Salvati E. Recurrent dislocation and the high-riding patella. Clin Orthop Relat Res 1972;88:67–9.
27. Cooney AD, Kazi Z, Caplan N, et al. The relationship between quadriceps angle and tibial tuberosity-trochlear groove distance in patients with patellar instability. Knee Surg Sports Traumatol Arthrosc 2012;20(12):2399–404.
28. Merchant AC. Patellofemoral imaging. Clin Orthop Relat Res 2001;(389): 15–21.
29. Dejour D, Le Coultre B. Osteotomies in patello-femoral instabilities. Sports Med Arthrosc 2007;15(1):39–46.
30. Barnett AJ, Prentice M, Mandalia V, et al. Patellar height measurement in trochlear dysplasia. Knee Surg Sports Traumatol Arthrosc 2009;17(12):1412–5.
31. Berg EE, Mason SL, Lucas MJ. Patellar height ratios. A comparison of four measurement methods. Am J Sports Med 1996;24(2):218–21.

32. Seil R, Muller B, Georg T, et al. Reliability and interobserver variability in radiological patellar height ratios. Knee Surg Sports Traumatol Arthrosc 2000;8(4): 231–6.
33. Dejour H, Walch G, Nove-Josserand L, et al. Factors of patellar instability: an anatomic radiographic study. Knee Surg Sports Traumatol Arthrosc 1994;2(1): 19–26.
34. Lippacher S, Dejour D, Elsharkawi M, et al. Observer agreement on the Dejour trochlear dysplasia classification: a comparison of true lateral radiographs and axial magnetic resonance images. Am J Sports Med 2012;40(4):837–43.
35. Dye SF, Chew MH. The use of scintigraphy to detect increased osseous metabolic activity about the knee. Instr Course Lect 1994;43:453–69.
36. Elias DA, White LM, Fithian DC. Acute lateral patellar dislocation at MR imaging: injury patterns of medial patellar soft-tissue restraints and osteochondral injuries of the inferomedial patella. Radiology 2002;225(3):736–43.
37. Camp CL, Stuart MJ, Krych AJ, et al. CT and MRI measurements of tibial tubercle-trochlear groove distances are not equivalent in patients with patellar instability. Am J Sports Med 2013;41(8):1835–40.
38. Maenpaa H, Lehto MU. Patellar dislocation. The long-term results of nonoperative management in 100 patients. Am J Sports Med 1997;25(2):213–7.
39. Buchner M, Baudendistel B, Sabo D, et al. Acute traumatic primary patellar dislocation: long-term results comparing conservative and surgical treatment. Clin J Sport Med 2005;15(2):62–6.
40. Palmu S, Kallio PE, Donell ST, et al. Acute patellar dislocation in children and adolescents: a randomized clinical trial. J Bone Joint Surg Am 2008;90(3):463–70.
41. Dolak KL, Silkman C, Medina McKeon J, et al. Hip strengthening prior to functional exercises reduces pain sooner than quadriceps strengthening in females with patellofemoral pain syndrome: a randomized clinical trial. J Orthop Sports Phys Ther 2011;41(8):560–70.
42. Cowan SM, Bennell KL, Crossley KM, et al. Physical therapy alters recruitment of the vasti in patellofemoral pain syndrome. Med Sci Sports Exerc 2002;34(12): 1879–85.
43. Cowan SM, Bennell KL, Hodges PW. Therapeutic patellar taping changes the timing of vasti muscle activation in people with patellofemoral pain syndrome. Clin J Sport Med 2002;12(6):339–47.
44. Smith TO, Donell ST, Chester R, et al. What activities do patients with patellar instability perceive makes their patella unstable? Knee 2011;18(5):333–9.
45. Hughston JC, Deese M. Medial subluxation of the patella as a complication of lateral retinacular release. Am J Sports Med 1988;16(4):383–8.
46. Fithian DC, Paxton EW, Post WR, et al. Lateral retinacular release: a survey of the International Patellofemoral Study Group. Arthroscopy 2004;20(5):463–8.
47. Halbrecht JL. Arthroscopic patella realignment: an all-inside technique. Arthroscopy 2001;17(9):940–5.
48. Nam EK, Karzel RP. Mini-open medial reefing and arthroscopic lateral release for the treatment of recurrent patellar dislocation: a medium-term follow-up. Am J Sports Med 2005;33(2):220–30.
49. Boddula MR, Adamson GJ, Pink MM. Medial reefing without lateral release for recurrent patellar instability: midterm and long-term outcomes. Am J Sports Med 2014;42(1):216–24.
50. Miller JR, Adamson GJ, Pink MM, et al. Arthroscopically assisted medial reefing without routine lateral release for patellar instability. Am J Sports Med 2007; 35(4):622–9.

51. Sillanpaa PJ, Maenpaa HM, Mattila VM, et al. Arthroscopic surgery for primary traumatic patellar dislocation: a prospective, nonrandomized study comparing patients treated with and without acute arthroscopic stabilization with a median 7-year follow-up. Am J Sports Med 2008;36(12):2301–9.
52. Sillanpaa PJ, Mattila VM, Maenpaa H, et al. Treatment with and without initial stabilizing surgery for primary traumatic patellar dislocation. A prospective randomized study. J Bone Joint Surg Am 2009;91(2):263–73.
53. Schottle PB, Scheffler SU, Schwarck A, et al. Arthroscopic medial retinacular repair after patellar dislocation with and without underlying trochlear dysplasia: a preliminary report. Arthroscopy 2006;22(11):1192–8.
54. Ahmad CS, Stein BE, Matuz D, et al. Immediate surgical repair of the medial patellar stabilizers for acute patellar dislocation. A review of eight cases. Am J Sports Med 2000;28(6):804–10.
55. Camp CL, Krych AJ, Dahm DL, et al. Medial patellofemoral ligament repair for recurrent patellar dislocation. Am J Sports Med 2010;38(11):2248–54.
56. Christiansen SE, Jakobsen BW, Lund B, et al. Isolated repair of the medial patellofemoral ligament in primary dislocation of the patella: a prospective randomized study. Arthroscopy 2008;24(8):881–7.
57. Sallay PI, Poggi J, Speer KP, et al. Acute dislocation of the patella. A correlative pathoanatomic study. Am J Sports Med 1996;24(1):52–60.
58. Mountney J, Senavongse W, Amis AA, et al. Tensile strength of the medial patellofemoral ligament before and after repair or reconstruction. J Bone Joint Surg Br 2005;87(1):36–40.
59. Csintalan RP, Latt LD, Fornalski S, et al. Medial patellofemoral ligament (MPFL) reconstruction for the treatment of patellofemoral instability. J Knee Surg 2014; 27(2):139–46.
60. Deie M, Ochi M, Adachi N, et al. Medial patellofemoral ligament reconstruction fixed with a cylindrical bone plug and a grafted semitendinosus tendon at the original femoral site for recurrent patellar dislocation. Am J Sports Med 2011; 39(1):140–5.
61. Dopirak R, Adamany D, Bickel B, et al. Reconstruction of the medial patellofemoral ligament using a quadriceps tendon graft: a case series. Orthopedics 2008;31(3):217.
62. Drez D Jr, Edwards TB, Williams CS. Results of medial patellofemoral ligament reconstruction in the treatment of patellar dislocation. Arthroscopy 2001;17(3):298–306.
63. Farr J, Schepsis AA. Reconstruction of the medial patellofemoral ligament for recurrent patellar instability. J Knee Surg 2006;19(4):307–16.
64. Fisher B, Nyland J, Brand E, et al. Medial patellofemoral ligament reconstruction for recurrent patellar dislocation: a systematic review including rehabilitation and return-to-sports efficacy. Arthroscopy 2010;26(10):1384–94.
65. Goyal D. Medial patellofemoral ligament reconstruction: the superficial quad technique. Am J Sports Med 2013;41(5):1022–9.
66. He W, Yang YM, Liu M, et al. Reconstruction of the medial patellofemoral ligament using hamstring tendon graft with different methods: a biomechanical study. Chin Med Sci J 2013;28(4):201–5.
67. Howells NR, Barnett AJ, Ahearn N, et al. Medial patellofemoral ligament reconstruction: a prospective outcome assessment of a large single centre series. J Bone Joint Surg Br 2012;94(9):1202–8.
68. Panagopoulos A, van Niekerk L, Triantafillopoulos IK. MPFL reconstruction for recurrent patella dislocation: a new surgical technique and review of the literature. Int J Sports Med 2008;29(5):359–65.

69. Schottle P, Schmeling A, Romero J, et al. Anatomical reconstruction of the medial patellofemoral ligament using a free gracilis autograft. Arch Orthop Trauma Surg 2009;129(3):305–9.
70. Schottle PB, Fucentese SF, Romero J. Clinical and radiological outcome of medial patellofemoral ligament reconstruction with a semitendinosus autograft for patella instability. Knee Surg Sports Traumatol Arthrosc 2005;13(7):516–21.
71. Elias JJ, Cosgarea AJ. Technical errors during medial patellofemoral ligament reconstruction could overload medial patellofemoral cartilage: a computational analysis. Am J Sports Med 2006;34(9):1478–85.
72. Beck P, Brown NA, Greis PE, et al. Patellofemoral contact pressures and lateral patellar translation after medial patellofemoral ligament reconstruction. Am J Sports Med 2007;35(9):1557–63.
73. Shah JN, Howard JS, Flanigan DC, et al. A systematic review of complications and failures associated with medial patellofemoral ligament reconstruction for recurrent patellar dislocation. Am J Sports Med 2012;40(8):1916–23.
74. Tanaka MJ, Bollier MJ, Andrish JT, et al. Complications of medial patellofemoral ligament reconstruction: common technical errors and factors for success: AAOS exhibit selection. J Bone Joint Surg Am 2012;94(12):e87.
75. Servien E, Fritsch B, Lustig S, et al. In vivo positioning analysis of medial patellofemoral ligament reconstruction. Am J Sports Med 2011;39(1):134–9.
76. McCarthy M, Ridley TJ, Bollier M, et al. Femoral tunnel placement in medial patellofemoral ligament reconstruction. Iowa Orthop J 2013;33:58–63.
77. Fulkerson JP. The effects of medialization and anteromedialization of the tibial tubercle on patellofemoral mechanics and kinematics. Am J Sports Med 2007;35(1):147 [author reply: 148].
78. Mihalko WM, Boachie-Adjei Y, Spang JT, et al. Controversies and techniques in the surgical management of patellofemoral arthritis. Instr Course Lect 2008;57:365–80.
79. Pidoriano AJ, Weinstein RN, Buuck DA, et al. Correlation of patellar articular lesions with results from anteromedial tibial tubercle transfer. Am J Sports Med 1997;25(4):533–7.
80. Barber FA, McGarry JE. Elmslie-Trillat procedure for the treatment of recurrent patellar instability. Arthroscopy 2008;24(1):77–81.
81. Cosgarea AJ, Schatzke MD, Seth AK, et al. Biomechanical analysis of flat and oblique tibial tubercle osteotomy for recurrent patellar instability. Am J Sports Med 1999;27(4):507–12.
82. Stetson WB, Friedman MJ, Fulkerson JP, et al. Fracture of the proximal tibia with immediate weightbearing after a Fulkerson osteotomy. Am J Sports Med 1997;25(4):570–4.
83. Fulkerson JP. Fracture of the proximal tibia after Fulkerson anteromedial tibial tubercle transfer. A report of four cases. Am J Sports Med 1999;27(2):265.
84. Koh JL, Ko D. Fulkerson anteromedialization osteotomy. Tech Knee Surg 2009;8(2):104–9.
85. Buuck DA, Fulkerson JP. Anteromedialization of the tibial tubercle: a 4- to 12-year follow-up. Oper Tech Sports Med 2000;8:131–7.
86. Duncan ST, Noehren BS, Lattermann C. The role of trochleoplasty in patellofemoral instability. Sports Med Arthrosc 2012;20(3):171–80.
87. Dejour D, Saggin P. The sulcus deepening trochleoplasty–the Lyon's procedure. Int Orthop 2010;34(2):311–6.
88. Goutallier D, Raou D, Van Driessche S. Retro-trochlear wedge reduction trochleoplasty for the treatment of painful patella syndrome with protruding trochleae.

Technical note and early results. Rev Chir Orthop Reparatrice Appar Mot 2002; 88(7):678–85 [in French].

89. Peterson LA, Vasiliadis HS. Proximal open trochleoplasty (grooveplasty), in patellofemoral pain, instability, and arthritis. In: Zattagnini S, DeJour D, Arendt EA, editors. Berlin, Heidelberg (Germany): Springer-Verlag; 2010. p. 217–24.

90. Donell ST, Joseph G, Hing CB, et al. Modified Dejour trochleoplasty for severe dysplasia: operative technique and early clinical results. Knee 2006;13(4): 266–73.

91. Faruqui S, Bollier M, Wolf B, et al. Outcomes after trochleoplasty. Iowa Orthop J 2012;32:196–206.

92. Blond L, Schottle PB. The arthroscopic deepening trochleoplasty. Knee Surg Sports Traumatol Arthrosc 2010;18(4):480–5.

Management of Patellofemoral Chondral Injuries

Adam B. Yanke, MD*, Thomas Wuerz, MD,
Bryan M. Saltzman, MD, Davietta Butty, BS, Brian J. Cole, MD, MBA

KEYWORDS

- Articular cartilage • Patellofemoral • Autologous chondrocyte implantation
- Osteochondral allograft • Microfracture • Patellofemoral chondral defects
- Tibial tubercle osteotomy • Articular cartilage techniques

KEY POINTS

- Proper clinical indications is the keystone to successful outcomes in patellofemoral cartilage lesion treatment.
- Overlooking an unloading or realignment osteotomy may lead to clinical failure.
- There is limited data to recommend microfracture of the patellofemoral joint.
- Improved reliability in surgical treatment is seen with: low BMI, pain for less than a year, objective effusions, and no prior surgery.

INTRODUCTION: NATURE OF THE PROBLEM

Patients can develop patellofemoral pain for several reasons, including acute trauma and overuse injuries. The underlying cause may be rooted in a chondral defect. In the professional athlete, the prevalence of patellofemoral defects was 37%, with 64% of these being patellar.[1] Similar findings have been described in patients undergoing routine knee arthroscopy, with patellar lesions present in 36% of knees.[2]

Despite the relatively high prevalence of incidental lesions, no data exist to support prophylactic treatment. Although chondral lesions may progress in size,[3] clinicians should focus on short-term improvement in patient symptoms, including objective findings, such as swelling.

Department of Orthopedic Surgery, Rush University Medical Center, 1611 W Harrison Street, Chicago, IL 60612, USA
* Corresponding author.
E-mail address: basworth@mac.com

Clin Sports Med 33 (2014) 477–500
http://dx.doi.org/10.1016/j.csm.2014.03.004
0278-5919/14/$ – see front matter © 2014 Elsevier Inc. All rights reserved.

sportsmed.theclinics.com

Although patellofemoral defects are commonly associated with valgus malalignment or patellar instability, this review focuses on the treatment of the defect itself. Associated osteotomies and their role are also included; however, the general treatment of patellar dislocations is not covered.

HISTORY

Successful treatment hinges on accurate diagnosis, which can be obtained from a thorough history and physical examination. Factors that can modify patient outcome are workers' compensation status, and previous surgery. Body mass index (BMI, calculated as weight in kilograms divided by the square of height in meters) may not have the same role in progression of patellofemoral defects as it does in tibiofemoral defects.[4] Typically, patients complain of anterior knee pain that is deep to the patella, and patients gesture with 1 finger to the patella or describe a band inferior to the patella adjacent to the infrapatellar fat pad. Trochlear lesions can also cause posterior knee pain. Symptoms are exacerbated by going down stairs, which requires the most knee flexion of activities of daily living. Stairs also place the largest load on the patellofemoral joint, causing symptom flares. Running, jumping, kneeling, and squatting also exacerbate pain. Patients also describe the movie theater sign, in which anterior knee pain is increased after prolonged sitting. Symptoms are typically not worsened with walking on level ground.

Although these are classic symptoms, a history of knee swelling and symptoms caused by a traumatic event is more focal and indicates a true lesion. The duration of pain should be evaluated, because patients with more acute onset and shorter duration of symptoms are more likely to have predictable pain relief. Catching, popping, or clicking that is not associated with true mechanical symptoms or pain isolated to these events are nonspecific and unlikely to be addressed successfully with surgery.

If the patient has a history of patellar instability, the clinician should be diligent to determine if pain and discomfort are present when the knee is stable or only when dislocation/subluxation events occur. If it is the former, there is a possibility that a chondral defect is the culprit. However, our preference is not to treat lesions that are found incidentally in patients with symptoms related only to instability events. This history is not always clear; therefore, using a patellar stabilization brace can aid patients in determining if instability is the inciting factor. Similarly, a positive yet transient response to an intra-articular injection can correlate with improved response to foretell the response that a patient might have to a cartilage procedure.

Nonoperative management should include injections and bracing, as discussed earlier. However, the mainstay of treatment is physical therapy, which includes quadriceps strengthening, peripatellar mobilization, core strengthening, abductor strengthening, and physiotaping. Antiinflammatories in conjunction with an injection can also decrease the effect of the inflammatory cascade. This treatment should be continued for 6 weeks to 6 months, depending on the patient's response. Continued pain in the setting of normal range of motion and symmetric thigh circumference are concerning for failure of nonoperative management.

PHYSICAL EXAMINATION

- General
  - Gait (antalgic, Trendelenburg, in-toeing)
  - Lower extremity alignment

- Q angle (anterior superior iliac spine–central patella–tibial tuberosity): male: 14 ± 3°, female: 17 ± 3°[5]
  - Measure at 0° and 30° of flexion when patella is engaged in the trochlea
- Femoral anteversion
- Inspection
  - Patellar tracking with flexion and extension
  - If J sign is present, determine at what degree of flexion it occurs
    - Hold medializing force on the patella during knee range of motion to determine if improved symptoms of instability
      - Improvement of symptoms is most likely related to medial patellofemoral ligament laxity opposed to lateral contracture[6]
  - Vastus medialis atrophy and thigh circumference difference
- Palpation
  - Joint effusion
  - Patellar tilt, translation, and apprehension
  - Patellar grind test and crepitus
  - Decreased range of motion
  - Iliotibial band contracture
  - Provocative maneuvers (deep squat, laterally directed patellar force with knee range of motion)

INDICATIONS/CONTRAINDICATIONS

Indications and contraindications are listed in **Boxes 1–4**.

SURGICAL TECHNIQUE/PROCEDURE

- Preoperative planning
  - Radiographs
    - Standing anteroposterior, Rosenberg posteroanterior (45° of flexion), lateral and sunrise or Merchant view (45°–60° of flexion)
    - 30° flexion views of the patellofemoral joint are best to assess patellar maltracking and condylar dysplasia
    - Lateral view to asses for patella alta (Blumensaat line, Blackburn-Peel, or Insall-Salvati methods)
    - Standing mechanical axis in the setting of instability
  - Advanced imaging
    - Magnetic resonance imaging (MRI)

Box 1
General indications for cartilage restoration

- Characteristic anterior knee pain
- Pain not always associated with instability
- Failure of aggressive nonsurgical management
- Joint effusions
- Corresponding lesion on radiographs with possible bone marrow edema
- Positive response to injection even if temporary
- Outerbridge grade III to IV lesion

Box 2
Relative contraindications for cartilage restoration

- Increased BMI
- Worker's compensation
- Significant bone marrow edema at the time of surgery
- Radiographic evidence of joint space narrowing (Kellgren Lawrence grade III–IV)

- Axial T1 and T2 useful for detecting effusions and to evaluate the patello-femoral chondral surface
- Axial T2 evaluation for subchondral edema
- Axial view for trochlear dysplasia or lateral patellar facet prominence
- The TT-TG distance can be measured on axial views, with normal being ~15 mm and 50% of patients with symptomatic patellofemoral disease have TT-TG greater than 20 mm, whereas this is true in only 5% of asymptomatic knees (**Fig. 1**)[7]
- Sagittal views aid in determining proximal/distal aspect of the lesion and evaluation of the suprapatellar pouch for loose bodies
- Determine presence of acute chondral or osteochondral fragment associated with patellar dislocation
- Remainder is important to rule out any concomitant disease
  - Computed tomography
    - Similar to MRI, the TT-TG distance can be measured on axial views
- Preparation and patient positioning
  ○ Supine on operating table
  ○ Bump placed under the operative hip is optional based on alignment
  ○ Tourniquet (we prefer to use throughout the procedure)
- Surgical approach
  ○ Arthroscopy should be performed using an inferolateral and inferomedial para-patellar portal with an optional outflow portal
    - Because these lesions are rarely treated primarily unless debridement or microfracture is performed, arthroscopy should be performed first for appropriate staging and possible cartilage biopsy
  ○ Three incisions can be chosen based on the likelihood of an isolated cartilage procedure, isolated osteotomy, or combined treatment (**Fig. 2**)
    - Incision is based centrally parallel to the tibial crest from the proximal pole of the patella to the 5 to 7 cm distal to the tibial tuberosity

---

Box 3
Indications for tibial tubercle (TT) osteotomy

- Symptomatic patellar or bipolar lesion
- Lateral or central patellar defect
- Direct anteriorization for isolated central/medial defect
- Patellar instability with increased TT–trochlear groove (TG) distance
- Patella alta
- Failed primary cartilage procedure with proper indication/technique

Box 4
Guidelines for specific cartilage procedures

Debridement

- Large flap component
- Not indicated for incidental lesions
- Lesions staged to undergo autologous chondrocyte implantation (ACI)

Microfracture

- Low demand
- Unipolar (trochlea>>patella)
- Lesion size less than 2 to 3 cm^2
- Augmentation of other cartilage procedures

Osteochondral allograft/autograft

- High demand
- Lesion size smaller than 3 cm^2 or lesions larger than 3 cm^2 with bone loss
- Revision of failed cartilage procedure

Cell-based cartilage therapies (ACI [Carticel, Genzyme, Cambridge, MA], DeNovo NT [Zimmer, Warsaw, IN])

- Lesion size greater than 3 cm^2 without bone loss
- Bipolar lesions are a relative contraindication
- Minimal bone marrow edema at time of treatment

- o We prefer a lateral versus medial arthrotomy
  - ■ Increased ability to access the patellofemoral joint without entering the quadriceps (vastus lateralis relatively more proximal than the vastus medialis)
  - ■ The arthrotomy is closed only proximal to the superior pole of the patella to act as a lateral release

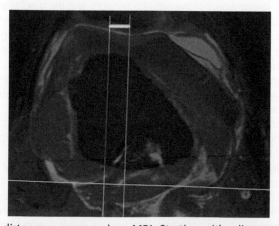

Fig. 1. The TT-TG distance as measured on MRI. Starting with a line perpendicular to the posterior condylar axis, a second line is drawn parallel to this through the TG. The distance between these 2 lines (*yellow line*) represents the TT-TG distance.

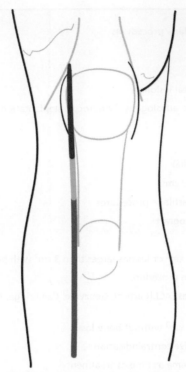

Fig. 2. The lateral-based skin incision for the surgical approach to address isolated cartilage lesions (*blue*), isolated osteotomy (*purple*), or both (*entire line*). The actual deep arthrotomy can be undermined up to the muscle belly of the vastus lateralis to aid in patellar eversion.

- ○ Dissection for combined osteotomy and cartilage treatment
- ○ Superficial dissection
- ○ The skin incision is made sharply, with soft tissue flaps developed above the fascia both medially and laterally, with adequate exposure to the tibial crest, the medial and lateral extent of the patellar tendon, and the medial and lateral portion of the patella, if a medial imbrication and lateral arthrotomy are to be performed
- ○ The fascia is then incised over the anterior compartment along the lateral crest of the tibia with a Bovie and continued proximally along the lateral aspect of the patellar tendon (**Fig. 3**)
  - ■ If the osteotomy is performed in conjunction with a cartilage procedure, this is carried proximally to the vastus lateralis to allow for patellar eversion or trochlear access
- ○ Use a Bovie to release the tissue medial to the patellar tendon and continue this distally until it converges at the tip of the osteotomy fragment, leaving a periosteal hinge
- ○ Use a Kelly clamp to ensure that the patellar tendon is freely mobile
- • Deep dissection
  - ○ The anterior compartment is then elevated off the tibia subperiosteally so that the posterior aspect of the tibia can be palpated with the surgeon's finger
    - ■ Depending on the osteotomy system used, the surgeon should ensure that a retractor such as a Chandler can fit to protect the neurovascular bundle (anterior tibial artery and deep peroneal nerve)

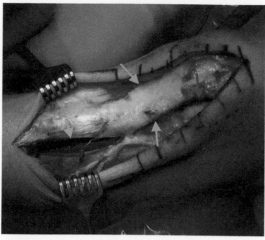

Fig. 3. Superficial dissection to perform both open cartilage restoration procedure and osteotomy. The arthrotomy is created laterally (*red arrow*), with the patellar tendon being freed both medially and laterally (*green arrows*). Distally, the fascia to the anterior compartment is released (*blue arrow*).

- Plan for the osteotomy to exit near the ridge anterior to the posterior aspect of the tibia
- Osteotomy
  - If performed in conjunction with a cartilage procedure, osteotomy should be performed first to aid in eversion of the patella
  - The exact technique of osteotomy formation varies based on the system used; here, the Arthrex (Naples) T3 system is discussed
    - Regardless of the system, most allow either a guide-based or freehand 45°, 60°, or 90° cut
    - We prefer the 60° cut in almost all instances to allow for 1 mm of medialization for every 2 mm of elevation
    - Typically, the osteotomy is translated 1 cm
  - Using a guide pin placed through the tibial tuberosity and perpendicular to the extremity long axis, the guide is used to prepare the osteotomy location
    - The proximal portion of the guide should start at the medial aspect of the patellar tendon, with the distal aspect just medial to the anterior aspect of the tibial crest
  - The jig should be provisionally fixed, and the osteotomy is performed with careful attention to prevent exit posterior to the tibia (**Fig. 4**)
    - Some systems allow for placement of a drill bit before osteotomy creation to ensure that the exit point is anterior to the posterior aspect of the tibia
    - The cuts should be made through the cortical portion of the tibia distally, with the proximal, metaphyseal portion finished with an osteotome
    - All attempts should be made to leave a distal hinge intact for osteotomy rotation
  - After the cartilage restoration procedure is completed, this can be provisionally fixed with a Kirschner wire and final fixation is performed with either 2 4.5-mm or 3 3.5-mm cortical screws
    - Care should be taken to use proper Arbeitsgemeinschaft für Osteosynthesefragen (AO) technique and countersink the screw heads to decrease prominence and decrease the chance of requiring a screw removal later

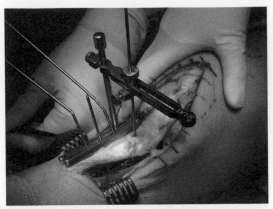

Fig. 4. The TT osteotomy is performed with the initial guide pin placed through the TT. The alignment arm (in this case set to 90°) is then attached to aid in placement of the cutting block.

- o Any prominent osseous ridge medial or lateral should be filed or sawed so there is no prominence
  - ◾ Sterile bone wax can be used for a similar purpose and to decrease bleeding
  - ◾ The tourniquet should be deflated at this point if used to control bleeding
- • Cartilage restoration procedure
  - o Microfracture
    - ◾ Equipment: microfracture awl or drill, curette
    - ◾ Microfracture can be performed through an open or arthroscopic technique; if performed arthroscopically, care should be taken that angled awls are available to allow for perpendicular access to the subchondral bone
    - ◾ The defect should initially be defined by removing all remaining diseased cartilage to the level of the calcified cartilage layer; this can be performed with a combination of a scalpel and curette; care should be taken to create vertical borders around the periphery of the defect of healthy hyaline articular cartilage
    - ◾ The calcified cartilage should then be removed, with care taken not to penetrate the subchondral bone
    - ◾ Using a microfracture awl or drill, the subchondral bone is penetrated, starting at the periphery of the defect, moving centrally, with 2 to 3 mm between perforations; care should be taken not to cause fracture of the region of the subchondral bone between microfracture sites (**Fig. 5**)
    - ◾ After completion, the inflow can be let down to ensure that subchondral bleeding is present from the microfracture sites
  - o ACI (second generation)
    - ◾ ACI requires 2 separate procedures, with the initial procedure involving harvest of 200 to 300 μg of full-thickness cartilage from the intercondylar notch for expansion (6–12 weeks)
    - ◾ Performed though an open exposure, the patellar or trochlear defect should be prepared as in the microfracture protocol with regard to creating vertical walls at the periphery and debridement of the calcified cartilage layer
    - ◾ The surgeon should ensure that no bleeding is present at this stage with the tourniquet down; if there is bleeding, fibrin glue can be pressed into the defect to decrease bleeding

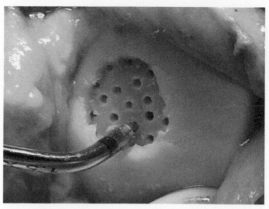

Fig. 5. Patellar microfracture as performed with a drill. Note the well-defined, vertical walls, with even spacing of the microfracture holes.

- First-generation ACI required usage of a periosteal patch, which resulted in a 30% reoperation rate; this has been improved with off-label usage of a type I/III synthetic collagen patch (Bio-Gide; Geistlich Pharma AG, Wolhusen, Switzerland); although we use this method in clinical practice, it cannot officially be recommended because of lack of US Food and Drug Administration approval
  - One vial of cells can be placed on the patch before insertion to allow chondrocyte adherence
  - The patch should be sewn to the periphery using a 6-0 Vicryl on a cutting needle (Ethicon, Somerville, NJ) spaced evenly (approximately 2 mm apart)
  - Care should be taken not to penetrate the patch multiple times for a given suture, and the needle should be passed from the patch to the cartilage
  - Leaving a small opening at the superior portion of the patch, place fibrin glue at the periphery of the patch; after this dries, place a small angiocatheter with a saline-filled syringe to test for a watertight seal and add sutures or fibrin where any deficiencies are present
  - Then use the angiocatheter to inject the remaining cells under the patch, followed by a final suture and fibrin glue layer (**Fig. 6**)
  - DeNovo NT (Zimmer)
    - Usage of DeNovo NT, an off-the-shelf source of particulated juvenile articular cartilage, can also be used in the setting of an Outerbridge grade III/IV of the trochlea or patella
    - The defect is prepared in a similar fashion to ACI before the patch is placed
    - At this stage, the DeNovo NT tissue is mixed with fibrin glue and placed in the defect site (**Fig. 7**)
  - Osteochondral allograft
    - Equipment: Arthrex osteochondral allograft tray, open orthopedic tray, pulsatile lavage irrigation
    - Perform standard parapatellar arthrotomy
    - Size the defect by placing the cylindrical guide over the defect
    - Mark the 12 o'clock position with a marking pen
    - Place guide pin through the cylinder guide and penetrate 2 cm

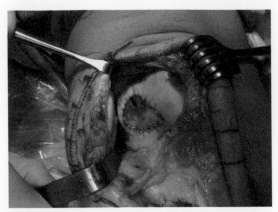

Fig. 6. The finished ACI construct as seen in the trochlea. Note the even spacing of the sutures, with the knots placed on the patch surface. Tension across the patch should be uniform and no dog-ears should be present.

- Remove sizing cylinder and ream with the corresponding size to 6 to 8 mm, decreasing allogeneic load
- Using a small ruler, measure the depth of the hole at 3, 6, 9, and 12 o'clock positions to allow contouring of the allograft to ensure that the graft is not proud or recessed
- Prepare the donor graft using an appropriately sized coring reamer in a similar manner to the recipient site preparation
- After plug removal, adjust the depth of the plug to match the clockface measurements
- The graft is then irrigated with pulsatile lavage to flush out bone marrow elements

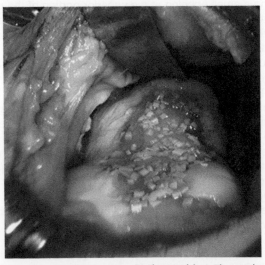

Fig. 7. DeNovo performed in an open manner in the trochlea. The explants are secured with fibrin glue, which is allowed to set before closure.

- Insert the donor plug in a press-fit manner with an oversized tamp
- Err on the side of more frequent, lighter taps, and do not leave the graft proud

COMPLICATIONS AND MANAGEMENT

TT osteotomy
- Symptomatic hardware (removal rate as high as 50%)[8]
- Infection
- Nonunion (increased BMI, smokers, obese)
- Fracture[9]
- Wound complications
- Compartment syndrome
- Peroneal nerve injury
- Deep vein thrombosis

Microfracture
- Intralesional osseous overgrowth
- Possibly obviates further cell-based technology

ACI
- Periosteal patch hypertrophy in first-generation ACI (**Fig. 8**)

DeNovo NT
- No specific complications

Osteochondral autograft
- Donor site morbidity
- Cyst formation

Osteochondral allograft
- Disease transmission
- Graft resorption

POSTOPERATIVE CARE

Postoperative care is outlined in **Table 1**.

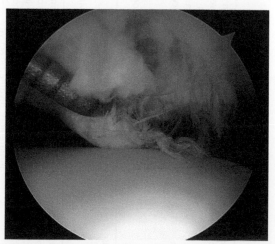

Fig. 8. First-generation ACI was plagued with a second operation rate of about 30% secondary to patch hypertrophy.

Table 1
Patellofemoral cartilage procedure rehabilitation

	Therapeutic Exercise	WB Without AMZ	WB with AMZ	Brace	Range of Motion
Phase I (0–6 wk)	1–6 wk: quad sets, SLR, hamstring isometrics; complete exercises in brace if quad control is inadequate	WB as tolerated	0–6 wk: heel touch with WB (20%)	0–1 wk: locked in full extension (removed for CPM and exercises) 2–4 wk: gradually open brace in 20° increments as quad control is gained; discontinue use of brace when quads can control SLR without an extension lag	0–6 wk: CPM, use for 6–8 h/d; begin at 0°–40°, increasing 5°–10° daily per patient comfort Patient should gain 100° by week 6
Phase II (6–12 wk)	6–10 wk: begin isometric closed chain exercises. At 6–10 wk, may begin weight-shifting activities with involved leg extended if full WB. At 8 wk, begin balance activities and stationary bicycle with light resistance 10–12 wk: hamstring strengthening, theraband 0°–30° resistance, light open chain knee isometrics		6–8 wk: transition to full WB	None	Gain full pain-free motion
Phase III (12 wk–6 mo)	Begin treadmill walking at a slow to moderate pace Progress balance/proprioceptive activities, initiate sport cord lateral drills	WB as tolerated			
Phase IV (6–9 mo)	Advance closed chain strengthening, initiate unilateral closed chain exercises, progress to fast walking and backward walking on treadmill (initiate incline at 8–10 mo), initiate light plyometric activity				
Phase V (9–12 mo)	Continue strength training, emphasize single leg loading, begin a progressive running and agility program. High-impact activities may begin after 12 mo if no swelling or pain				

Abbreviations: AMZ, anteromedialization; CPM, continuous passive motion; SLR, straight leg raise; WB, weight bearing.

OUTCOMES
Microfracture

In an evidence-based systematic review, Mithoefer and colleagues[10] evaluated 28 studies describing 3122 patients who had microfracture surgery for articular cartilage injury in the knee The average postoperative follow-up was 41 ± 5 months (range, 12–136) with an average age of 39 ± 10 years (range, 24–65) and an average lesion size of 3.0 ± 0.8 cm^2 (range, 0.1–20). None of the studies evaluated microfracture results specifically for patellofemoral cartilage defects only. Nineteen of the 28 studies reported on knees with both femorotibial and patellofemoral chondral defects. Microfracture improved knee function in all studies during the first 24 months after surgery. Improvement in knee function was reported in 67% to 86% of patients at an average of 6 to 7 years after surgery. Although 2 studies reported maintained outcomes after 2 years, 7 studies reported deterioration of initial functional improvement in 47% to 80% of patients between 18 and 36 months after the procedure (still better than preoperative). Younger patients, with threshold age varying between 30 and 40 years, resulted in better clinical outcome scores and better repair cartilage fill on MRI. The procedure was also more effective when used as a first-line procedure. These investigators concluded that microfracture provides effective short-term functional improvement of knee function, with limited hyaline repair tissue and possible deterioration over time.[10]

Microfracture was found to be a successful option for the treatment of full-thickness cartilage lesions of the knee (medial or lateral femoral condyle, trochlear, or patella) in a meta-analysis by Negrin and colleagues.[11] These investigators mentioned how numerous publications on microfracture show deterioration over time and that microfracture is ineffective for the treatment of large chondral lesions, better in patients younger than 35 years, and superior for lesions of the femoral condyles than of the patella.

When interpreting the outcomes of microfracture in the patellofemoral joint, it is important to remember that surgical technique plays a large role as well as to address concomitant factors. We believe that microfracture, compared with other cartilage techniques, is performed more frequently in isolation for defects that require concomitant osteotomy, unfairly biasing microfracture outcome data.

ACI

ACI has evolved since its inception, when it was first described using a periosteal patch.[12] Subsequent iterations have been termed as generations. Because this terminology is confounding through the literature, we define each generation as follows: first, covered with periosteal patch, second, covered with synthetic membrane, third, seeded onto a three-dimensional scaffold.[13]

Outcomes of patients with patellar chondral defects treated with first-generation, second-generation, or third-generation ACI were reported by Niemeyer and colleagues.[14] These investigators reported that patients aged 34.3 ± 10.1 years with 4.41 ± 2.15 cm^2 defects had favorable outcomes at 38.4 ± 15.6 months with regard to Lysholm and International Knee Documentation Committee (IKDC) scales. Eighty-four percent of patients believed that their symptoms were better after the operation, with 2.9% feeling the same and 12.9% saying their symptoms were worse. Defects located on the lateral facet had improved outcomes compared with other regions. Trochlear lesions treated with first-generation ACI by Mandelbaum and colleagues[15] showed an improvement in pain and swelling at a mean of 59 months. Of these patients, 43% were receiving workers' compensation. Data are conflicting regarding the effect of previous cartilage procedures on ACI outcome; however, we have not noticed this effect regarding first-generation ACI of the patellofemoral joint.[16] Long-term follow-up of first-generation ACI of the patellofemoral joint at an average of 12.6 years showed maintained improvement of Lysholm and Tegner scores.[17] In this study, although age was not predictive of outcome, kissing lesions had inferior results.

With regard to second-generation ACI, Vanlauwe and colleagues[18] reported that 84% of patients with patellofemoral joint lesions had clinically relevant improvement. Similarly, third-generation ACI of the patellofemoral joint has also yielded promising results at 5 years with the added benefit of arthroscopic implementation.[19] Subset analysis performed by Kreuz and colleagues[20] looked at third-generation ACI in the context of gender and defect location to determine if either influenced the results of the procedure. These investigators determined that all groups (males/females with condylar or patellofemoral defects) improved their clinical scores over the follow-up period; however, the cohort with the worst results was female patients with patellar defects. A retrospective matched-pair analysis compared 10 patients who underwent CaReS technique (third-generation ACI) with those treated with microfracture for patellofemoral lesions ($\sim$3 cm^2).[21] Although the CaReS ACI cohort improved at 36 months, this was not significantly different from the microfracture cohort.

As clinical results of first-generation, second-generation, and third-generation ACI continue to be reported, it is difficult to determine true superiority without adequate randomized controlled trials. In the meantime, systematic reviews have reported marginal improvement of second and third generation over first generation, but longer-term follow-up is necessary.[13]

Osteotomy

The role of the TT osteotomy has long been researched in the setting of patellofemoral disease. Several individual reports have specifically reported improved outcomes in combination with first-generation[8,16,22] and third-generation ACI compared with ACI alone.[23]

Trinh and colleagues[24] performed a systematic review of the literature to compare clinical outcomes of patients undergoing isolated patellofemoral ACI and ACI combined with patellofemoral realignment. Their report included 11 studies (10 level III or IV evidence), with a mean 4.2 years of follow-up, having 78% of defects located on the patella and 23% of which underwent previous or concomitant osteotomy (anteriorization, medialization, or anteromedialization). The ACI procedure was a first-generation procedure in 235 patients (64%) and a second-generation procedure in the remaining 131 patients (36%). Although significant improvements were observed in all studies, analysis showed that patients who underwent ACI and a TT unloading osteotomy had significantly greater improvements and absolute clinical scores (IKDC, Lysholm, Knee Injury and Osteoarthritis Outcome Score, Tegner score, modified Cincinnati score, Short Form 36 score, and Short Form 12 score) than those patients receiving ACI in isolation. Overall complication rates for isolated ACI patients was 15.2% (43 patients), which was not significantly less when compared with the 19% rate in patients undergoing previous or concomitant distal realignment procedures.

Because patients seem to have improved outcomes from the osteotomy aspect of surgery, it is reasonable to question to what extent the cartilage procedure affects the outcome. Atkinson and colleagues[25] reported on 50 isolated TT osteotomy procedures for Outerbridge III-IV defects. Twenty patients with a history of dislocation also received lateral trochlea elevation osteotomies. Ninety-four percent of knees had sustained significant improvement in visual analogue scales at mean 81 months follow-up, with 96% satisfied.

Although osteotomies have a clear role in improving the outcome of patellofemoral chondral defects, level I research is necessary to determine the true usefulness compared with the cartilage restoration procedure. We prefer distal realignment in patients with malalignment, instability, bipolar lesions, and all patellar lesions.

Osteochondral Autograft/Allograft Transplantation

Osteochondral autograft treatment of patellofemoral defects remains an option for salvage procedures and some primary lesions with bone loss (avascular necrosis/ osteochondritis dissecans/osteochondral defects).[26] Procedures performed for primary lesions of the patella (average 1.2 cm^2) evaluated 8 months postoperatively showed improved Lysholm scores.[27] Although MRI showed that the autograft surface was flush, 80% had mild bone marrow edema about the graft. Similarly, Karataglis and colleagues[28] reported 86.5% improvement of their preoperative symptoms. Although not performed frequently, osteochondral defects of the patella in patients not willing to undergo treatment with cadaveric tissue can successfully be treated with an osteo-chondral autograft.

Although limited literature exists on osteochondral allografts for the patellofemoral joint, a recent systematic review by Chahal and colleagues[29] described these outcomes compared with the tibiofemoral joint. Most studies used allografts for posttraumatic defects (38%), osteochondritis dissecans (30%), osteonecrosis from all causes (12%), and idiopathic (11%). With regards to the patellofemoral joint, these investigators concluded that diffuse lesions in this location treated with fresh osteochondral grafting show poorer results compared with lesions in the tibial plateau or femoral condyle.

Jamali and colleagues[30] analyzed osteochondral allograft treatment of the patellofemoral joint with improved pain, function, range of motion, and low risk of progressive arthritis. The high failure rate (25%) and revision surgery (53%) are likely caused by the size of the lesions treated (patella: 7.1 cm^2, range 1.8–17.8; trochlea 13.2 cm^2, range 2.5–22.5). Kaplan-Meier analysis showed a 67% ± 25% allograft survival probability at 10 years. Patellofemoral resurfacing with shell allografts has been reported by Torga Spak and Teitge.[31] These investigators reported a high failure rate (42%); however, patients who did not fail were satisfied and had improved subjective scores. Three grafts survived for more than 10 years.

Osteochondral allografts and autografts can be successful in unipolar patellofemoral lesions with bone loss in young patients (**Table 2**).

Patellofemoral Arthroplasty

Although not discussed in detail in this review, patellofemoral arthroplasty (PFA) remains an option as a primary procedure for radiographic patellofemoral arthritis or a salvage procedure for failed cartilage procedures. Because data for the latter are lacking, the outcomes of PFA for diffuse patellofemoral arthritis are reported. Data on PFA report that patients do well at 3 to 7 years with regard to pain relief and 88% survival, with 3.6% to 11.6% total knee arthroplasty (TKA) conversion rate.[32–34] Long-term follow-up of the Richards prosthesis at an average of 17 to 20 years showed 86% good to excellent results; however, this was tempered by a 44% rate of surgical revision for disease progression and 31% conversion rate to TKA.[35,36]

A systematic review of the literature on PFA was completed by Tarassoli and colleagues.[37] Poor outcomes were associated with evidence of tibiofemoral osteoarthritis before surgery, BMI greater than 30 kg/m^2, previous meniscectomy, patella

Table 2
Studies of patellofemoral chondral injuries

Procedure Citation	Study Design Cohort (Age, Previous Operation Number)	Defect Size	Follow-up	Results	Concluding Remarks
Microfracture Mithoefer et al,[10] 2009	Systematic review, 28 studies, N = 3122 Coleman Methodology Score: 58 Age 39 ± 10 y Lesions of trochlea, patella, MFC, LFC	Mean 3.0 ± 0.8 cm^2 (range 0.1–20 cm^2)	Mean 41 ± 5 mo (range 12–136 mo)	Knee function improved 67%–86% at 6–7 y Longest study: 32% pain free, 54% mild pain, 14% moderate pain (11 y follow/up) Failure/revision: 2.5% at 2 y, 23%–31% between 2–5 y (in 6 randomized controlled trails)	7 studies reported deterioration of initial functional improvement in 47%–80% between 18–36 mo postoperatively Age <30–40 y: better outcomes and MRI cartilage fill
Microfracture Negrin et al,[11] 2012	Meta-analysis, 5 studies, N = 187 Age 15–60 y	Range 1–10 cm^2	Range 2–5 y	Mean standardized treatment effect: 1.106 Expected increase of 22 overall KOOS points	Decreased outcomes after 18–24 mo Ineffective for treatment of large chondral lesions <35 y improved outcomes LFC/MFC outcomes superior to patella
First-generation ACI Mandelbaum et al,[15] 2007	Prospective cohort study, N = 40 43% workers' compensation Age 37.1 ± 8.5 y 78% previous surgery Lesions of trochlea	Mean 4.5 ± 2.8 cm^2	Mean 59 ± 18 mo	Significant improvements in condition score (3.1 ± 1.0 to 6.4 ± 1.7), pain (2.6 ± 1.7 to 6.2 ± 2.4), and swelling (3.9 ± 2.7 to 6.3 ± 2.7)	First-generation ACI adequately addresses pain, condition, and swelling in trochlear lesions

First-generation ACI Vasiliadis et al,[17] 2010	Retrospective cohort study, N = 92 Age 35 y (range, 14–57)	Mean 5.5 ± 2.9 cm²	Mean 12.6 ± 2.3 y	Median Tegner score = 2→3 (P<.05) Median Lysholm score = 61→70 (P>.05) 72% better or unchanged 93% would undergo the operation again Outcomes not affected by age or lesion size	One of the longest clinical follow-up studies for first-generation ACI 93% of patients would undergo surgery again
First-generation ACI Pascual-Garrido et al,[16] 2009	Prospective cohort study, N = 62 Age 31.8 y (range 15.8–49.4)	Mean 4.2 ± 1.6 cm²	Mean 4 y (range 2–7)	Significant improvement in Lysholm, IKDC, KOOS Pain, KOOS Symptoms, KOOS Activities of Daily Living, KOOS Sport, KOOS Quality of Life, SF-12 Physical, Cincinnati, and Tegner No significant improvement in SF-12 Mental 44% reoperation rate 7.7% failure rate (arthroplasty or conversion to osteochondral allograft)	Outcome was not affected by previous cartilage procedures Patients undergoing AMZ tended to have better outcomes
Second-generation ACI Vanlauwe et al,[18] 2012	Prospective cohort study, N = 38 Age 30.9 y Lesions of patella (28), trochlea (7), or both (3) 84% of patients had previous surgery	Mean 4.89 cm² (range 1.5–11 cm²)	Mean 37 mo (range 24–72 mo)	Significant improvements in KOOS and VAS at 48 mo 84% clinically relevant improvement >10 patients at 3 y 13% failure 24% reoperation	Second-generation ACI yields promising outcomes in the patellofemoral joint at 3 y

(continued on next page)

Table 2
(continued)

Procedure Citation	Study Design Cohort (Age, Previous Operation Number)	Defect Size	Follow-up	Results	Concluding Remarks
Third-generation ACI Gobbi et al,[19] 2009	Case series, N = 34 Age 31.2 y (range 15–55 y) Lesions of the patella (21), trochlea (9), or both (4)	Mean 4.45 cm²	5 y	Significant improvement in IKDC, VAS, and Tegner at 2 and 5 y	Third-generation ACI has good results in the patellofemoral joint at 5 y
Third-generation ACI Kreuz et al,[20] 2013	Comparison study (men vs women), N = 25 men; 27 women Age, 35.6 y 20 PF compartment lesions	Males: 7.00 ± 3.7 cm² Females: 4.33 ± 1.1 cm²	Follow-up at 6, 12, and 48 mo	Female PF lesions: Lysholm/IKDC improved at 6 mo, with continued IKDC improvement Male PF lesions: Lysholm/IKDC improved at 6 mo with significant improvement at 12 mo also	Male and female patients both improve after third-generation ACI for patellar defects; however, men have greater improvement
First-generation, second-generation, and third-generation ACI Niemeyer et al,[14] 2008	Retrospective study, N = 70 Age 34.3 ± 10.1 y Mean previous operations 1.55 ± 1.4	Mean 4.41 ± 2.15 cm²	Mean 38.4 ± 15.6 mo	Improved IKDC (61.6 ± 21.5), Lysholm (73.0 ± 22.4), and Cumulated Ambulation Score 61.5 ± 21.5 Symptoms better 84%, same 2.9%, and worse 12.9% 67% normal/nearly normal International Cartilage Repair Society 81.4% would have operation again	Patellar ACI yields good results in 70%–80% of patients

First-generation ACI ± AMZ (73.7% concomitant) Farr,[8] 2007	Prospective study, N = 39 (38 knees) Age 31.2 ± 11.3 y Patella and trochlea	Trochlea: 4.3 ± 1.9 cm^2 (46% of cohort) Patella: 5.4 ± 1.9 cm^2 (36% of cohort) Bipolar: 8.8 ± 3.5 cm^2 (18% of cohort)	Mean 1.2 y	Modified Cincinnati Overall Condition score: median 3-point improvement Lysholm score: median 31-point improvement VAS score resting: median 2-point improvement VAS score maximum: 3-point improvement 25 patients had 32 subsequent surgeries 3 patients failed ACI	Overall condition improved regardless of concurrent AMZ or presence of >1 lesion
First-generation ACI ± AMZ Henderson & Lavigne,[22] 2006	Comparison study, N = 22 per group, lesions of patella	N/A	Mean 2 y	Osteotomy with greater increase in mean modified Cincinnati Knee Score (4.5 vs 1.7 points), better function (1.7 vs 2.5), better SF-36 physical component scores (70.9 vs 55.4 points), higher IKDC scores (85.2 vs 60.6 points)	Patellar ACI with osteotomy has better outcomes than ACI alone, possibly in patient with normal PF biomechanics
Third-generation ACI + distal realignment Gigante et al,[23] 2009	Prospective cohort study, N = 14 knees (12 patients) Age 31 y	Median 4 cm^2 (range 3–9 cm^2)	Mean 3 y	Improved Modified Cincinnati and median Lysholm, Tegner, and Kujala Score 13/14 patients satisfied 50% excellent, 43% good, 7% poor final outcomes	93% of patients with third-generation ACI and osteotomy have good/ excellent results

(continued on next page)

Table 2
(continued)

Procedure Citation	Study Design Cohort (Age, Previous Operation Number)	Defect Size	Follow-up	Results	Concluding Remarks
TT advancement osteotomy ± medialization (50%) ± lateral trochlea elevation osteotomy (25%) Atkinson et al,[25] 2012	Retrospective cohort study, N = 40 Age 29 y (range 17–51 y)	N/A	Mean 81 mo (26–195 mo)	92%–96% satisfied and improved VAS and Shelbourne and Trumper anterior knee function scores 77% excellent/good, 35% fair, 8% poor 2 knees required arthroplasty (18 mo, 8 y) 12% major complications 8% superficial wound infections 44% hardware discomfort	TT osteotomy alone yields promising results at an average of 81 mo This study helps challenge the effect of the cartilage procedure, promoting the need for level I evidence for cartilage restoration with osteotomy
Osteochondral autograft transplantation Figueroa et al,[27] 2011	Retrospective cohort study, N = 10 Lesions of patella	Mean 1.2 cm²	N/A	Lysholm 73.8 ± 8.36 → 95 ± 4.47 IKDC postoperatively 95 ± 1.74 No postoperative complications MRI: no fissures in graft-receptor interface in 60%, mild bone marrow edema about the graft in 80%	Clinical outcomes scores and advanced imaging show that osteochondral autografts are a viable option for defects with bone loss
Osteochondral autograft transplantation Karataglis et al,[28] 2006	Case series, N = 37 knees Age 31.9 y (range 18–48 y) 26 femoral condyle, 11 patellofemoral joint	Mean 2.73 cm² (range 0.8–12 cm²)	Mean 36.9 mo (18–73 mo)	86.5% reported improvement in their preoperative symptoms and returned to previous occupation 48.6% returned to sports	Although no patellofemoral subset analysis was performed, no correlation was found with respect to lesion size or location

Study	Design	Lesion size	Follow-up	Results	Conclusions
Osteochondral allograft transplantation Chahal et al,[29] 2013	Systematic review, 19 studies; N = 644 knees Age 37 y (range 20–62 y) 20 trochlear and 45 patellar lesions	Mean 6.3 cm²	Mean 58 mo (range 19–120 mo)	Overall satisfaction rate 86% 65% showed little/no arthritis at final follow-up Short-term complication rate 2.4% Overall failure rate 18%	Osteochondral allografts have inferior results in the patellofemoral joint compared with tibiofemoral lesions
Osteochondral allograft transplantation Jamali et al,[30] 2005	Retrospective cohort study, N = 20 (18 patients) Age 42 y (range 19–64 y) 8 patellar and 12 trochlea/patella	Mean patella 7.1 cm² (range, 1.8–17.8 cm²) Mean trochlea 13.2 cm² (range 2.5–22.5 cm²)	Mean 94 mo (range 24–214 mo)	60% good/excellent 25% failure: revision allograft (2), total knee arthroplasty (2), arthrodesis (1) Radiographs (12 knees): no PF arthrosis (4), mild arthrosis (6) Kaplan-Meier analysis 67 ± 25% allograft survival probability at 10 y	Osteochondral allografts can yield promising results when successful; however, this study reported poor long-term survival in these large defects
Osteochondral allograft transplantation Torga Spak & Teitge,[31] 2006	Retrospective cohort study, N = 14 knees (11 patients) Age 37 y (range 24–56 y) Mean previous operations, 4.4 2 patellar and 12 patellofemoral	Shell PF grafts	Mean, 10 y (range, 2.5–17.5 y)	6/14 revised to arthroplasty 10 of 11 successes would have procedure again Knee Society Scores 46→82 Functional Scores 50→75 Lysholm 27→80 Mean extension lag 12°→3° Reoperation in 12 of 14 Complications in 4 patients (persistent anterior knee pain, skin rash)	Fresh osteochondral allografts for diffuse PF osteoarthritis can provide limited results, with a 42% failure rate Patients may benefit because of delay of arthroplasty

Abbreviations: AMZ, anteromedialization; IKDC, International Knee Documentation Committee; KOOS, Knee Injury and Osteoarthritis Outcome Score; LFC, Lateral Femoral Condyle; MFC, Medial Femoral Condyle; N/A, not applicable; PF, patellofemoral; SF, Short Form; VAS, visual analogue scale.

alta or baja, and ligamentous instability. The most common reason that they found cited for failure necessitating revision was progression of tibiofemoral osteoarthritis. However, it was concluded that PFA is a less invasive operation, with more rapid post-operative recovery and preservation of bone stock to allow for conversion to TKA at a later date.

SUMMARY

Treatment of patellofemoral chondral defects is fraught with difficulty because of the generally inferior outcomes and significant biomechanical complexity of the joint. Noyes and Barber-Westin[38] performed a systematic review of large (>4 cm^2) patello-femoral ACI (11 studies), PFA (5 studies), and osteochondral allografting (2 studies) in patients younger than 50 years. Respectively, failures or poor outcomes were noted in 8% to 60% after ACI, 22% after PFA, and 53% after osteochondral allograft treatment. As noted in the outcome reviews earlier, unacceptable complication and reoperation rates were reported from all 3 procedures, and it was concluded that each operation had unpredictable results for this patient demographic. This study highlights the importance of strict indications and working to address all concomitant diseases to decrease revision rate. Outcomes are most predictable in young patients with low BMI and unipolar defects lower than 4 cm^2.

REFERENCES

1. Flanigan DC, Harris JD, Trinh TQ, et al. Prevalence of chondral defects in athletes' knees: a systematic review. Med Sci Sports Exerc 2010;42:1795–801.
2. Widuchowski W, Widuchowski J, Trzaska T. Articular cartilage defects: study of 25,124 knee arthroscopies. Knee 2007;14:177–82.
3. Wang Y, Ding C, Wluka AE, et al. Factors affecting progression of knee cartilage defects in normal subjects over 2 years. Rheumatology (Oxford) 2006;45:79–84.
4. Ding C, Cicuttini F, Scott F, et al. Natural history of knee cartilage defects and factors affecting change. Arch Intern Med 2006;166:651–8.
5. Mihalko WM, Boachie-Adjei Y, Spang JT, et al. Controversies and techniques in the surgical management of patellofemoral arthritis. Instr Course Lect 2008;57: 365–80.
6. Cole BJ, Gomoll AH, Minas T, et al. Treatment of chondral defects in the patello-femoral joint. J Knee Surg 2006;19:285–95.
7. Dejour H, Walch G, Nove-Josserand L, et al. Factors of patellar instability: an anatomic radiographic study. Knee Surg Sports Traumatol Arthrosc 1994;2:19–26.
8. Farr J. Autologous chondrocyte implantation improves patellofemoral cartilage treatment outcomes. Clin Orthop Relat Res 2007;463:187–94.
9. Pidoriano AJ, Weinstein RN, Buuck DA, et al. Correlation of patellar articular lesions with results from anteromedial tibial tubercle transfer. Am J Sports Med 1997;25:533–7.
10. Mithoefer K, McAdams T, Williams RJ, et al. Clinical efficacy of the microfracture technique for articular cartilage repair in the knee: an evidence-based systematic analysis. Am J Sports Med 2009;37:2053–63.
11. Negrin L, Kutscha-Lissberg F, Gartlehner G, et al. Clinical outcome after micro-fracture of the knee: a meta-analysis of before/after-data of controlled studies. Int Orthop 2012;36:43–50.
12. Brittberg M, Lindahl A, Nilsson A, et al. Treatment of deep cartilage defects in the knee with autologous chondrocyte transplantation. N Engl J Med 1994;331: 889–95.

13. Goyal D, Goyal A, Keyhani S, et al. Evidence-based status of second- and third-generation autologous chondrocyte implantation over first generation: a systematic review of level I and II studies. Arthroscopy 2013;29:1872–8.
14. Niemeyer P, Steinwachs M, Erggelet C, et al. Autologous chondrocyte implantation for the treatment of retropatellar cartilage defects: clinical results referred to defect localisation. Arch Orthop Trauma Surg 2008;128: 1223–31.
15. Mandelbaum BR, Browne J, Fu F, et al. Treatment outcomes of autologous chondrocyte implantation for full-thickness articular cartilage defects of the trochlea. Am J Sports Med 2007;35:915–21.
16. Pascual-Garrido C, Slabaugh MA, L'Heureux DR, et al. Recommendations and treatment outcomes for patellofemoral articular cartilage defects with autologous chondrocyte implantation: prospective evaluation at average 4-year follow-up. Am J Sports Med 2009;37(Suppl 1):33S–41S.
17. Vasiliadis HS, Wasiak J, Salanti G. Autologous chondrocyte implantation for the treatment of cartilage lesions of the knee: a systematic review of randomized studies. Knee Surg Sports Traumatol Arthrosc 2010;18:1645–55.
18. Vanlauwe JJ, Claes T, Van Assche D, et al. Characterized chondrocyte implantation in the patellofemoral joint: an up to 4-year follow-up of a prospective cohort of 38 patients. Am J Sports Med 2012;40:1799–807.
19. Gobbi A, Kon E, Berruto M, et al. Patellofemoral full-thickness chondral defects treated with second-generation autologous chondrocyte implantation: results at 5 years' follow-up. Am J Sports Med 2009;37:1083–92.
20. Kreuz PC, Niemeyer P, Müller S, et al. Influence of sex on the outcome of autologous chondrocyte implantation in chondral defects of the knee. Am J Sports Med 2013;41:1541–8.
21. Petri M, Broese M, Simon A, et al. CaReS (MACT) versus microfracture in treating symptomatic patellofemoral cartilage defects: a retrospective matched-pair analysis. J Orthop Sci 2013;18:38–44.
22. Henderson IJ, Lavigne P. Periosteal autologous chondrocyte implantation for patellar chondral defect in patients with normal and abnormal patellar tracking. Knee 2006;13:274–9.
23. Gigante A, Enea D, Greco F, et al. Distal realignment and patellar autologous chondrocyte implantation: mid-term results in a selected population. Knee Surg Sports Traumatol Arthrosc 2009;17:2–10.
24. Trinh TQ, Harris JD, Siston RA, et al. Improved outcomes with combined autologous chondrocyte implantation and patellofemoral osteotomy versus isolated autologous chondrocyte implantation. Arthroscopy 2013;29:566–74.
25. Atkinson HD, Bailey CA, Anand S, et al. Tibial tubercle advancement osteotomy with bone allograft for patellofemoral arthritis: a retrospective cohort study of 50 knees. Arch Orthop Trauma Surg 2012;132:437–45.
26. Lu AP, Hame SL. Autologous osteochondral transplantation for simple cyst in the patella. Arthroscopy 2005;21:1008.
27. Figueroa D, Meleán P, Calvo R, et al. Osteochondral autografts in full thickness patella cartilage lesions. Knee 2011;18:220–3.
28. Karataglis D, Green MA, Learmonth DJ. Autologous osteochondral transplantation for the treatment of chondral defects of the knee. Knee 2006;13:32–5.
29. Chahal J, Cole BJ, Gross AE, et al. Outcomes of osteochondral allograft transplantation in the knee. Arthroscopy 2013;29:575–88.
30. Jamali AA, Emmerson BC, Chung C, et al. Fresh osteochondral allografts: results in the patellofemoral joint. Clin Orthop Relat Res 2005;(437):176–85.

31. Torga Spak R, Teitge RA. Fresh osteochondral allografts for patellofemoral arthritis: long-term followup. Clin Orthop Relat Res 2006;444:193–200.
32. Ackroyd CE, Chir B. Development and early results of a new patellofemoral arthroplasty. Clin Orthop Relat Res 2005;(436):7–13.
33. Leadbetter WB, Kolisek FR, Levitt RL, et al. Patellofemoral arthroplasty: a multicentre study with minimum 2-year follow-up. Int Orthop 2009;33(6):1597–601. http://dx.doi.org/10.1007/s00264-008-0692-y.
34. Mont MA, Johnson AJ, Naziri Q, et al. Patellofemoral Arthroplasty 7-year Mean Follow-Up. J Arthroplasty 2011. http://dx.doi.org/10.1016/j.arth.2011.07.010.
35. Kooijman HJ, Driessen APPM, van Horn JR. Long-term results of patellofemoral arthroplasty. A report of 56 arthroplasties with 17 years of follow-up. J Bone Joint Surg Br 2003;85(6):836–40.
36. van Jonbergen H-PW, Poolman RW, van Kampen A. Isolated patellofemoral osteoarthritis. Acta Orthop 2010;81(2):199–205. http://dx.doi.org/10.3109/1745367100 3628756.
37. Tarassoli P, Punwar S, Khan W, et al. Patellofemoral arthroplasty: a systematic review of the literature. Open Orthop J 2012;6(1):340–7. http://dx.doi.org/10.2174/1874325001206010340.
38. Noyes FR, Barber-Westin SD. Advanced patellofemoral cartilage lesions in patients younger than 50 years of age: is there an ideal operative option? Arthroscopy 2013;29:1423–36.

MPFL Reconstruction
Technique and Results

 CrossMark

Jeffrey Reagan, MD, Raj Kullar, MD, Robert Burks, MD*

KEYWORDS

- Medial patellofemoral ligament • Patellar instability • Patellar dislocation

KEY POINTS

- Preoperative evaluation for risk factors of patellar instability is warranted to identify contributing factors to instability apart from medial patellofemoral ligament (MPFL) pathology.
- The evaluation begins with examination of knee under anesthesia to confirm patellar instability.
- Diagnostic knee arthroscopy is performed to note morphology of trochlea, chondral injuries, and lateral displacement of the patella.
- During harvest of hamstring tendon, complete dissection of adhesions from semitendinosus should be ensured and damage to superficial medial collateral ligament should be avoided.
- Placement of patellar tunnel at the junction of the proximal and middle thirds of the patella is recommended.
- Risk of patellar fracture should be limited by drilling the patellar tunnel only to a depth of about 20 mm with sequential cleaning of the bit every few millimeters while using copious irrigation to limit thermal damage.
- It should be ensured that the patellar tunnel avoids violation of anterior cortex and subchondral bone.
- Femoral tunnel placement is aided by fluoroscopy on a true lateral view of the knee for anatomic graft position.
- Graft should be tunneled through the soft tissue in an extrasynovial manner in layer 2 of the knee.
- To avoid overconstraint by the graft, fixation should be done with the knee in 50° to 60° of flexion.
- This technique re-creates the neutralizing force on the patella; additional procedures may be needed if medicalization of the patella is desired to address lower limb malalignment.

 Video of an MPFL reconstruction with semitendinosis autograft accompanies this article at http://www.sportsmed.theclinics.com/

Disclosures: The authors report the following potential conflict of interest or source of funding. R. Burks receives support from Arthrex.
Department of Orthopaedics, University of Utah, 590 Wakara Way, Salt Lake City, UT 84108, USA
* Corresponding author.
E-mail address: Robert.Burks@hsc.utah.edu

INTRODUCTION

Dislocation of the patella represents 2% to 3% of all knee injuries.[1] The MPFL is nearly always injured with patellar dislocation and is the main restraint to lateral patellar translation.[2–12] Recurrent patellar instability may occur in 15% to 40% of patients who have been treated nonoperatively for first-time patellar dislocations.[13–15] This rate may increase up to 49% for patients who have had 2 prior patellar dislocations.[15] Recurrent instability episodes may lead to further cartilage injury, debilitating pain, and limitation of activities of daily living, and may limit return to sport.[12,16–18]

This subset of patients that continues to have instability episodes may have predisposing factors that contribute to patellar instability, which include:

- Femoral anteversion
- External tibial torsion
- Genu valgum
- Patellar dysplasia
- Trochlear dysplasia
- Patella alta
- Vastus medialis obliquus atrophy
- Pes planus
- Generalized hyperlaxity

Valgus malalignment of the knee results in an increased Q angle and increased laterally directed force on the patella. In kind, increased femoral anteversion and external tibial torsion results in rotational malalignment that may result in an increased lateral force vector to the patella and possible lateral subluxation. As the knee flexes, the proximal soft tissue restraints of the patella, including the MPFL, guide it into the trochlear groove.[3,4] In deep flexion, the bony constraints of the patellofemoral articulation provide stability. In patients with patella alta, this bony constraint occurs at a deeper flexion angle and can be more prone to dislocation or subluxation. In patients with trochlear dysplasia, the patellofemoral articulation yields insufficient constraint to lateral translation in flexion.[16]

For patients with traumatic causes of patellar instability, the MPFL tears (**Fig. 1**) and leads to loss of static restraint to lateral patellar translation. Injury of the MPFL may occur at the patellar origin, the femoral insertion, or the MPFL may sustain an intrasubstance tear. Injury may also occur at a combination of these sites.[4,19]

The goal of nonoperative treatment is to recondition and strengthen dynamic stabilizers of the patella.[20] In situations in which adequate therapy does not yield sufficient dynamic stabilization of the patella, reconstruction of the MPFL may be required. For patients who have failed nonoperative management, reconstruction of the MPFL is an accepted method to restore static medial stabilization.[21–25] For patients with other predisposing factors outlined earlier, further evaluation should be performed to determine the need for additional procedures to address the underlying abnormal anatomy and causes of recurrent subluxation.

Acute repair of the MPFL has been studied in the literature. With regard to primary patellar dislocation and acute MPFL injury, Camanho and colleagues[26] described 33 patients with a minimum of 25-months' follow-up. Of the 33 patients, 16 patients had nonoperative treatment with bracing and physical therapy and 8 had recurrent dislocations; 17 patients had MPFL repair and none had recurrent dislocations. All those who had MPFL repair had improved Kujala scores. Numerous other investigators, however, have not had as much success with acute repair.[27–30] Christiansen and colleagues[27] reported on 77 patients with 2-year follow-up in a randomized controlled trial. All patients had arthroscopy and then were randomized to MPFL repair versus

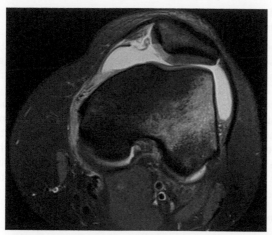

Fig. 1. T2 axial magnetic resonance image demonstrating a tear of the MPFL near the femoral insertion in a patient who had a lateral patellar dislocation. (*From* Wylie JD, Burks RT. Medial patellofemoral ligament reconstruction with semitendinosus autograft. Arthrosc Tech 2013;2(4):e418; with permission.)

nonoperative treatment. Of the total, 42 patients had MPFL repair with a 17% redislocation rate; 35 patients were treated in a nonoperative manner, and 20% of these had redislocation. In this group of patients, MPFL repair did not reduce the recurrence rate of dislocation and there were no improvements in the Kujala score.

Multiple studies have described MPFL reconstruction using anatomic and radiographic methods to obtain accurate tunnel placement.[7,8,22,31–35] Anatomic femoral and patellar tunnel placement is important in re-creating MPFL anatomy. If nonanatomic tunnel positions are used, then abnormal tension may be created, leading to increased patellofemoral contact pressures, pain with flexion or extension, early arthrosis, loosening or graft stretching, and recurrent instability.

INDICATIONS

With the reportedly high recurrence rate with nonoperative management, surgical intervention may be necessary. Numerous procedures to address patellofemoral instability have been described. Some of these include medial retinacular reefing and lateral release. These procedures can result in recurrent subluxation, continued knee pain, and iatrogenic medial instability.[36–39] The goal of reconstruction of the MPFL is to re-create a static medial restraint to lateral patellar translation while the knee is in extension and assist in guiding the patella into the trochlear groove.

The most common indication for MPFL reconstruction includes recurrent patellar instability with failed nonoperative management. Patients with chronic instability and trochlear dysplasia may also benefit from MPFL reconstruction.

CONTRAINDICATIONS

Contraindications to MPFL reconstruction are few. Systemic or local infection is an absolute contraindication. If MPFL reconstruction alone is performed when coexisting factors for instability exist, then there is a higher potential for graft failure. MPFL reconstruction should not be performed to pull or recenter the patella. In this clinical setting, addressing malalignment and malrotation in combination with MPFL reconstruction may be indicated.

SURGICAL TECHNIQUE
Preoperative Planning

Preoperatively, the patient's operative extremity should be assessed for previous surgeries, including scars or previous hamstring harvest. In addition, anteroposterior (AP), lateral, and merchant radiographs may be obtained to evaluate associated tibial tubercle malalignment or trochlear dysplasia.

Schöttle and colleagues[7] performed a cadaveric study describing a method of radiographic identification of the femoral insertion of the MPFL. To maintain isometry, a point within 5 mm of the anatomic MPFL femoral insertion should be used.[7,40] Redfern and colleagues[35] have shown that a fluoroscopically guided technique can accurately identify the anatomic origin of the MPFL, which is accomplished with a true lateral view of the distal femur and by identifying a point 0.5 mm anterior to the distal posterior cortex and 3 mm proximal to Blumensaat line.

Preparation and Patient Positioning

The patient should be positioned supine on a standard operating room table. After induction of general anesthesia, the knee is examined to confirm patellar laxity. A nonsterile tourniquet is then placed on the proximal thigh. A kidney post is placed laterally to assist with stability of the extremity with the knee at 90° flexion. The contralateral extremity is well padded to prevent undue pressure. AP and lateral fluoroscopic images should be taken before prepping and draping the extremity. The C-arm fluoroscopy unit should be positioned on the operative side, with the sterile table and instruments placed at the foot of the bed.

The operative extremity is prepared with ethanol followed by ChloraPrep (Care Fusion Corporation, San Diego, CA, USA). A down sheet is then placed under the limb, and the distal extremity placed in a stockinette with Coban wrap (3M, St Paul, MN, USA). Sterile U-drapes and an extremity drape complete the draping process.

Surgical Approach

Graft harvest

If an autograft is chosen, a 3- to 4-cm anteromedial incision is made over the proximal tibia at the level of the tibial tubercle at the midpoint in the sagittal plane. The semitendinosus is identified and bluntly dissected with a right-angle clamp. Blunt dissection is used to identify and develop the plane between the superficial medial collateral ligament (MCL) and the pes tendons. The semitendinosus is then released off the tibia and whipstiched with a #2 FiberWire suture (Arthrex, Inc, Naples, FL, USA). Traction is applied to the tendon, and adhesions are released with Metzenbaum scissors, until the muscle belly of the semitendinosus can be easily palpated. The tendon is stripped with a tendon stripper. Graft diameter is a typically 4 to 5 mm in size. The pes anserine is then closed with 0 Vicryl suture, and subcutaneous tissues are closed with 3-0 monocryl suture.

Patellar preparation

A 2- to 3-cm incision is made along the medial border of the patella (**Fig. 2**). A full-thickness subperiosteal flap including the MPFL and medial retinaculum are elevated off the proximal third of the patella in an extrasynovial, extra-articular manner.

With this exposure, the C-arm is brought in and a perfect lateral radiograph is obtained to localize the junction between the proximal and middle thirds of the patella. A guidewire is then placed at this point and drilled approximately 25 mm into the patella (**Fig. 3**). C-arm images are taken to confirm that the patella is drilled in appropriate dimensions in both the coronal and sagittal planes to avoid cortical or articular penetration (**Fig. 4**). A 5-mm cannulated drill bit (Arthrex MPFL Convenience Pack) is used

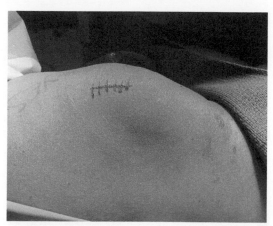

Fig. 2. A 2- to 3-cm medial patellar incision is made for placement of the patellar tunnel. The incision is made just lateral to the medial patella to allow for elevation of a full-thickness flap off the patella. (*From* Wylie JD, Burks RT. Medial patellofemoral ligament reconstruction with semitendinosus autograft. Arthrosc Tech 2013;2(4):e418; with permission.)

to drill a tunnel of at least 20 mm in the patella. The drill bit has small flutes, so it is important to ream in a staged manner, removing the reamer to clean the flutes and proceeding slowly with ample irrigation to minimize heat necrosis. The edges of the tunnel are curetted to allow for easy passage of the graft (**Fig. 5**).

Femoral preparation

Fluoroscopic imaging is used to obtain a perfect lateral image of the knee. A radiolucent marker is used to identify a point, or the radiographic intersection of the posterior femoral cortical line and Blumensaat line as described by Redfern and colleagues,[35] which represents most closely the anatomic insertion of the MPFL. A 2- to 3-cm skin incision is then made, and subcutaneous tissues are dissected with care taken

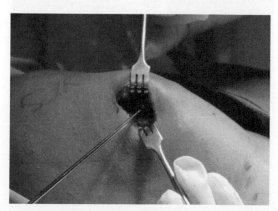

Fig. 3. A guide pin is placed at the junction of the upper and middle thirds of the patella at adequate depth to avoid cortical or intra-articular penetration. (*From* Wylie JD, Burks RT. Medial patellofemoral ligament reconstruction with semitendinosus autograft. Arthrosc Tech 2013;2(4):e418; with permission.)

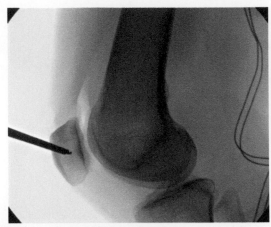

Fig. 4. A fluoroscopic lateral image of the knee is taken to confirm placement of the guide-wire for proper drilling of the tunnel at the middle and superior thirds of the patella. (*From* Wylie JD, Burks RT. Medial patellofemoral ligament reconstruction with semitendinosus autograft. Arthrosc Tech 2013;2(4):e418; with permission.)

to avoid injury to the saphenous nerve. A beath pin is then placed at this point under radiographic guidance and then drilled in a posterior to anterior direction through the femur and out of the lateral skin (**Fig. 6**). A cannulated 6- or 7-mm bit (based on graft sizing) is then passed to a distance of 40 to 45 mm into the femur (**Fig. 7**). The reamer is then removed, and a passing suture is shuttled using the beath pin.

Graft passage
A hemostat clamp is used to develop an extrasynovial tunnel from the patellar incision to the medial femoral incision. This process can be aided by dissecting the margin of the patella and developing a plane in layer 2 of the knee, superficial to capsule. It is important to not penetrate through the capsule into the joint. A passing suture is then passed from the medial femoral to the patellar incision to be ready for graft passage.

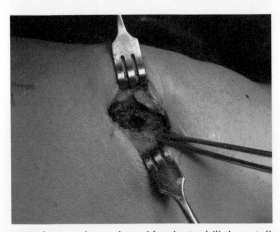

Fig. 5. A 5-mm reamer is then used over the guide wire to drill the patella to a depth of only about 20 mm. Soft tissues are cleared to allow graft passage into the patellar tunnel. (*From* Wylie JD, Burks RT. Medial patellofemoral ligament reconstruction with semitendinosus autograft. Arthrosc Tech 2013;2(4):e418; with permission.)

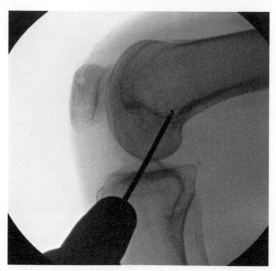

Fig. 6. A fluoroscopic lateral image of the knee with the drill bit placed at the point described by Redfern and colleagues[35] to localize drilling of the femoral tunnel. (*From* Wylie JD, Burks RT. Medial patellofemoral ligament reconstruction with semitendinosus autograft. Arthrosc Tech 2013;2(4):e419; with permission.)

The semitendinosus graft is first fixed into the patella. The whipstitched end of the graft is then threaded through a 4.75- or 5.5-mm docking anchor (SwiveLock, Arthrex, Inc) and secured so that approximately 15 mm of graft is pulled into the patellar tunnel. The docking anchor (SwiveLock, Arthrex, Inc) has an associated nonabsorbable braided suture, and this is retained for later closure of the retinaculum (**Fig. 8**).

The graft's free end is then tunneled to the femoral incision using the passage suture (**Fig. 9**). The free end is then cut to appropriate length and whipstitched with a #2 Vicryl

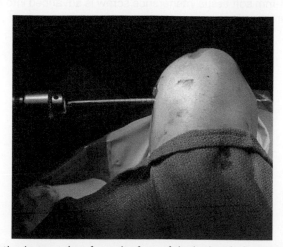

Fig. 7. Intraoperative image taken from the foot of the bed with the reamer advanced over the guide pin engaging the medial side of the femur. Drilling of the femoral tunnel is performed from medial (*left*) to lateral (*right*). The guide pin can be seen exiting the lateral thigh (*right*). (*From* Wylie JD, Burks RT. Medial patellofemoral ligament reconstruction with semitendinosus autograft. Arthrosc Tech 2013;2(4):e419; with permission.)

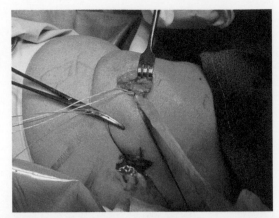

Fig. 8. The semitendinosus graft is fixed into the patellar tunnel. Passing stitches are in position for tunneling the graft to the femoral incision (*bottom*) in an extrasynovial manner through layer 2 of the knee. (*From* Wylie JD, Burks RT. Medial patellofemoral ligament reconstruction with semitendinosus autograft. Arthrosc Tech 2013;2(4):e419; with permission.)

suture, measuring enough graft to advance approximately 30 mm into the femoral tunnel. The #2 Vicryl suture ends are then looped into the passing stitch and are subsequently pulled through the femoral tunnel. The Vicryl suture ends are pulled to advance the graft into the femoral tunnel. At this point, mild tension is placed on the graft, and the knee is brought through its range of motion to assess the graft. The patella is checked to ensure there is adequate but not excessive tension on the graft. The patella should be easily translated at least 1 quadrant with a firm endpoint and dislocation prevented. The goal here is to remove the slack from the graft, but to avoid tensioning the graft.

A nitinol wire is then advanced into the femoral tunnel to guide screw placement. With the slack removed from the graft, and the knee at 50° to 60° of flexion, a 6 × 23-mm or 7 × 23-mm soft tissue interference screw is advanced into the femoral tunnel until good purchase is obtained.

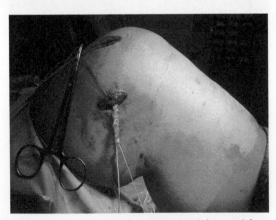

Fig. 9. The graft has been passed through the extrasynovial tunnel from the patellar origin to the femoral insertion site. The free graft end has been whipstitched and is ready to be passed into the femoral tunnel. The knee is flexed to 50° to 60° in preparation for final graft fixation. (*From* Wylie JD, Burks RT. Medial patellofemoral ligament reconstruction with semitendinosus autograft. Arthrosc Tech 2013;2(4):e419; with permission.)

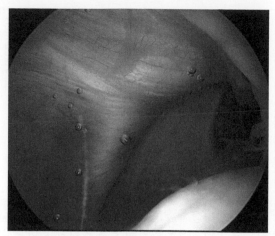

Fig. 10. The extra-articular semitendinosus graft used to reconstruct the MPFL can be seen with the arthroscope from a standard anterolateral knee portal. (*From* Wylie JD, Burks RT. Medial patellofemoral ligament reconstruction with semitendinosus autograft. Arthrosc Tech 2013;2(4):e420; with permission.)

An arthroscope is then placed into the knee to confirm that the patella sits centrally on the trochlea and that the graft is in an extra-articular position (**Fig. 10**). Arthroscopy can also precede MPFL reconstruction if the surgeon desires to evaluate the initial patellar position and assess the pathologic condition.

The nonabsorbable braided suture from the patellar tunnel docking anchor (Swive-Lock, Arthrex, Inc) is used to close the medial patellar retinaculum. Soft tissues are closed with monofilament suture, and the skin, in a subcuticular manner. Soft dressings are applied, and the knee is placed in a knee immobilizer.

Table 1	
MPFL reconstruction postoperative protocol	
0–3 wk postop	Motion, advance as tolerated WBAT in brace immobilizer Quad sets, 4-way hip exercises, calf raises Discontinue immobilizer with return of quad control
3–5 wk postop	Motion, advance as tolerated WBAT with crutches or one crutch for support Continue with quad sets, 4-way hip, and calf raises
5–6 wk postop	Motion full ROM Stationary bike with minimal resistance and then progress as tolerated Can begin closed-chain double-leg strengthening exercises as tolerated
6–12 wk postop	Continue with full A/PROM Continue with closed-chain double-leg strengthening as tolerated Start running when capable
12–16 wk postop	May progress to closed-chain single-leg strengthening as tolerated May begin functional exercises as tolerated Gradual return to sport

Abbreviations: AROM, active ROM; postop, postoperative; PROM, passive ROM; ROM, range of motion; WBAT, weight bear as tolerated.

Table 2
Results of MPFL reconstruction for recurrent patellar instability

Author, Year	Age	Knees	Follow-Up (y)	Graft Type	Redislocation	Subluxation	Apprehension	Outcome Measures	Other Complications	Combined Procedures
Deie et al,[42] 2003	8.5	6	7.4	ST	0	0	2	Kujala 96.3		
Deie et al,[43] 2005	19.2	46	5	ST	0	4	4	Kujala <50/>90		4 VMOA, 39 VMOA & LR
Deie et al,[31] 2011	22.2	31	3.2	ST	0	0	1	Kujala 64/94.5		
Drez et al,[24] 2001	22	15	2.6	GA, ST, or fascia lata	0	1	0	Kujala 88.6, Tegner 6.7, Fulkerson 93% good to excellent		
Ellera Gomes et al,[44] 2004	26.7	16	3.3	ST	0	1	1	Crosby-Insall 15/16 good to excellent, Aglietti 14/16 good to excellent		
Fernandez et al,[45] 2005	30	30	3.2	ST	0	0	0	Larsen and Lauridsen 29/30 good to excellent	Superficial wound infection 1/30	
Hinterwimmer et al,[46] 2013	19	19	1.3	GA	0	0	—	Kujala 92, Tegner 5, 89% patient satisfaction	0.16	
Kohn et al,[47] 2013	22	42	2	GA	0	0	—	Kujala 51/85, Tegner 2.4/4.9, IKDC 50/80, 87% satisfaction		17 reclosures of LR, 4 retransfers of TT, 5 distal femur osteotomies, 1 trochleoplasty
Mikashima et al,[48] 2006	21.8	24	2	ST	0	0	1	Kujala 30.5/95.5	2 patellar fractures	

Study	Age	N	F/U	Graft				Outcome	Complications	Reoperations
Nomura & Inoue,[21] 2006	24.8	12	4.2	ST	0	0	0	Kujala 56.3/96, Insall 83% good to excellent		3 LR
Raghuveer & Mishra,[49] 2012	29.2	15	3.5	ST or GA	0	0	2	Kujala 44.8/91.9, good to excellent 13/15	PF pain 2/15, external lag 1/15, Hardware pain 2/15	2 LR
Schöttle et al,[50] 2005	30.1	15	4	ST	0	2	4	Kujala 53.3/85.7, 88% good to excellent, 86% satisfaction		8 MTTO
Slenker et al,[51] 2013	20.6	35	1.75	12 Hamstring autografts, 23 hamstring allografts	0	0	0	Kujala 49.0/89.5		
Steiner et al,[52] 2006	27	34	5.5	23 Adductor tendon autografts, 6 bone-quad autografts, 5 bone-patellar tendon allografts	0	0	1	Kujala 53.3/90.7, Lysholm 52.4/92.1, Tegner 3.1/5.1, 91% good to excellent	1 hematoma, 1 traumatic loosening, 3 painful hardware removals	
Thaunat & Erasmus,[53] 2007	22	23	2.3	GA	0	0	0	Kujala 93	1 extension lag 10 degrees at final visit	
Toritsuka et al,[54] 2011	23	20	2.5	ST	1	0	1	Kujala 96, Crosby-Insall 6/20 excellent, 14/20 good		4 LR & ORIF of avulsion
Watanabe et al,[55] 2008	19	42	4.3	ST or GA	0	0	8	Lysholm >90		13 MTTO

Abbreviations: GA, gracilis autograft; LR, lateral release; MTTO, medial tibial tubercle osteotomy; ORIF, open reduction internal fixation; PF, patellofemoral; ST, semitendinosus autograft; VMOA, vastus medialis obliquus advancement.

POSTOPERATIVE CARE

The patient is sent home with the knee placed in a knee immobilizer to assist in pain control and quad control issues. Sutures are removed at the first postoperative visit, at which point radiographs are obtained to evaluate tunnel placement and to confirm no perioperative fracture. A continuous passive motion machine at home is allowed if desired. No range of motion restriction is needed. The immobilizer can aid with ambulation and may be discontinued when good quad control returns.

Physical therapy is started immediately postoperatively, with motion advanced as tolerated (**Table 1**). The patient is allowed to bear weight as tolerated in extension with the immobilizer. Return to sports is generally allowed around 3 to 4 months after surgery.

COMPLICATIONS AND MANAGEMENT

Numerous complications that occur with MPFL reconstruction involve patient selection errors and technical errors. These are factors that clinicians can limit with complete evaluation for anatomic factors that may contribute to patellar instability and by understanding the potential complications of MPFL reconstruction.

- Arthrofibrosis
- Infection
- Neurovascular injury (saphenous vein, saphenous nerve)
- Patellar fracture
- Recurrent lateral instability
- Patellofemoral arthritis
- Iatrogenic medial instability
- Painful hardware

Steps can be taken intraoperatively to minimize risks. Patellar fracture can lead to loss of graft fixation and increased morbidity for the patient. For this technique, the patellar tunnel is small in diameter (5 mm) and short (20–25 mm) to minimize stress riser. The technique of sequential drilling can also be helpful to minimize thermal injury to the bone. This process is aided by the use of new drill bits and by drilling only a few millimeters at a time, sequentially cleaning the drill bit during the tunnel reaming process.

Overtensioning of the graft can have significant consequences; it can cause altered patellofemoral contact pressures, which may lead to pain and arthrosis.[41] To avoid overtensioning, the knee should be flexed to 50° to 60° so that the patella is constrained within the trochlear groove, which provides a bony constraint to overtensioning because the patella is locked in the trochlear groove. The graft is not pulled to get it tight, but rather the slack is removed from the graft with the knee in this flexed position. It is also important to be aware of prior or concurrent lateral release because this may facilitate overconstraint medially.

OUTCOMES

The results of isolated MPFL reconstruction for recurrent patellar instability are promising. There are numerous retrospective case series studies showing successful prevention of recurrent dislocation or subluxation. Good to excellent results are reported in 80% to 96% of these reports. A summary of results is provided in **Table 2**.

The technique described is one method of MPFL reconstruction. This technique is performed in a minimally invasive manner, and its sure fixation allows for early motion and rehabilitation. This technique restores the main anatomic restraint to lateral patellar translation. However, a limitation of this technique is that it is not designed to functionally medialize the patella. If other predisposing factors to patellar instability exist, then MPFL reconstruction alone may not be sufficient and other procedures may be needed to address lower limb alignment, patella alta, and other abnormal anatomic factors.

SUMMARY

MPFL reconstruction is a viable option for treating patients with recurrent patellar instability, in whom nonoperative methods have failed to provide relief. It is important to evaluate patients for predisposing factors for patellar instability. This technique of MPFL reconstruction uses a reliable method to obtain anatomic tunnel position. Rigid fixation with interference fit in bone tunnels allows early range of motion and rehabilitation and minimizes concern for graft failure.

SUPPLEMENTARY DATA

Supplementary data related to this article can be found online at http://dx.doi.org/10.1016/j.csm.2014.03.006.

REFERENCES

1. Stefancin JJ, Parker RD. First-time traumatic patellar dislocation: a systematic review. Clin Orthop Relat Res 2007;455:93–101.
2. Amis AA, Firer P, Mountney J, et al. Anatomy and biomechanics of the medial patellofemoral ligament. Knee 2003;10(3):215–20.
3. Burks RT, Desio SM, Bachus KN, et al. Biomechanical evaluation of lateral patellar dislocations. Am J Knee Surg 1998;11(1):24–31.
4. Desio SM, Burks RT, Bachus KN. Soft tissue restraints to lateral patellar translation in the human knee. Am J Sports Med 1998;26(1):59–65.
5. Farr J, Schepsis AA. Reconstruction of the medial patellofemoral ligament for recurrent patellar instability. J Knee Surg 2006;19(4):307–16.
6. Sillanpää PJ, Peltola E, Mattila VM, et al. Femoral avulsion of the medial patellofemoral ligament after primary traumatic patellar dislocation predicts subsequent instability in men: a mean 7-year nonoperative follow-up study. Am J Sports Med 2009;37(8):1513–21.
7. Schöttle PB, Schmeling A, Rosenstiel N, et al. Radiographic landmarks for femoral tunnel placement in medial patellofemoral ligament reconstruction. Am J Sports Med 2007;35(5):801–4.
8. Stephen JM, Lumpaopong P, Deehan DJ, et al. The medial patellofemoral ligament: location of femoral attachment and length change patterns resulting from anatomic and nonanatomic attachments. Am J Sports Med 2012;40(8):1871–9.
9. Steensen RN, Dopirak RM, Maurus PB. A simple technique for reconstruction of the medial patellofemoral ligament using a quadriceps tendon graft. Arthroscopy 2005;21(3):365–70.
10. Weber-Spickschen TS, Spang J, Kohn L, et al. The relationship between trochlear dysplasia and medial patellofemoral ligament rupture location after patellar dislocation: an MRI evaluation. Knee 2011;18(3):185–8.
11. Parikh SN, Wall EJ. Patellar fracture after medial patellofemoral ligament surgery: a report of five cases. J Bone Joint Surg Am 2011;93(17):e97(1-8).
12. Sillanpää P, Mattila VM, Iivonen T, et al. Incidence and risk factors of acute traumatic primary patellar dislocation. Med Sci Sports Exerc 2008;40(4):606–11.

13. Mehta VM, Inoue M, Nomura E, et al. An algorithm guiding the evaluation and treatment of acute primary patellar dislocations. Sports Med Arthrosc 2007; 15(2):78–81.
14. Trikha SP, Acton D, O'Reilly M, et al. Acute lateral dislocation of the patella: correlation of ultrasound scanning with operative findings. Injury 2003;34(8):568–71.
15. Fithian DC, Paxton EW, Stone ML, et al. Epidemiology and natural history of acute patellar dislocation. Am J Sports Med 2004;32(5):1114–21.
16. Bollier M, Fulkerson J, Cosgarea A, et al. Technical failure of medial patellofemoral ligament reconstruction. Arthroscopy 2011;27(8):1153–9.
17. Bitar AC, Demange MK, D'Elia CO, et al. Traumatic patellar dislocation: nonoperative treatment compared with MPFL reconstruction using patellar tendon. Am J Sports Med 2012;40(1):114–22.
18. Colvin AC, West RV. Patellar instability. J Bone Joint Surg Am 2008;90(12): 2751–62.
19. Guerrero P, Li X, Patel K, et al. Medial patellofemoral ligament injury patterns and associated pathology in lateral patella dislocation: an MRI study. Sports Med Arthrosc Rehabil Ther Technol 2009;1(1):17.
20. McConnell J. Rehabilitation and nonoperative treatment of patellar instability. Sports Med Arthrosc 2007;15(2):95–104.
21. Nomura E, Inoue M. Hybrid medial patellofemoral ligament reconstruction using the semitendinous tendon for recurrent patellar dislocation: minimum 3 years' follow-up. Arthroscopy 2006;22(7):787–93.
22. Nomura E, Inoue M. Surgical technique and rationale for medial patellofemoral ligament reconstruction for recurrent patellar dislocation. Arthroscopy 2003; 19(5):E47.
23. Hautamaa PV, Fithian DC, Kaufman KR, et al. Medial soft tissue restraints in lateral patellar instability and repair. Clin Orthop Relat Res 1998;349:174–82.
24. Drez D Jr, Edwards TB, Williams CS. Results of medial patellofemoral ligament reconstruction in the treatment of patellar dislocation. Arthroscopy 2001;17(3): 298–306.
25. Sandmeier RH, Burks RT, Bachus KN, et al. The effect of reconstruction of the medial patellofemoral ligament on patellar tracking. Am J Sports Med 2000; 28(3):345–9.
26. Camanho GL, Viegas Ade C, Bitar AC, et al. Conservative versus surgical treatment for repair of the medial patellofemoral ligament in acute dislocations of the patella. Arthroscopy 2009;25(6):620–5.
27. Christiansen SE, Jakobsen BW, Lund B, et al. Isolated repair of the medial patellofemoral ligament in primary dislocation of the patella: a prospective randomized study. Arthroscopy 2008;24(8):881–7.
28. Palmu S, Kallio PE, Donell ST, et al. Acute patellar dislocation in children and adolescents: a randomized clinical trial. J Bone Joint Surg Am 2008;90(3):463–70.
29. Nikku R, Nietosvaara Y, Kallio PE, et al. Operative versus closed treatment of primary dislocation of the patella. Similar 2-year results in 125 randomized patients. Acta Orthop Scand 1997;68(5):419–23.
30. Nikku R, Nietosvaara Y, Aalto K, et al. Operative treatment of primary patellar dislocation does not improve medium-term outcome: a 7-year follow-up report and risk analysis of 127 randomized patients. Acta Orthop 2005;76(5):699–704.
31. Deie M, Ochi M, Adachi N, et al. Medial patellofemoral ligament reconstruction fixed with a cylindrical bone plug and a grafted semitendinosus tendon at the original femoral site for recurrent patellar dislocation. Am J Sports Med 2011; 39(1):140–5.

32. Panagopoulos A, van Niekerk L, Triantafillopoulos IK. MPFL reconstruction for recurrent patella dislocation: a new surgical technique and review of the literature. Int J Sports Med 2008;29(5):359–65.
33. Schottle PB, Romero J, Schmeling A, et al. Technical note: anatomical reconstruction of the medial patellofemoral ligament using a free gracilis autograft. Arch Orthop Trauma Surg 2008;128(5):479–84.
34. Servien E, Fritsch B, Lustig S, et al. In vivo positioning analysis of medial patellofemoral ligament reconstruction. Am J Sports Med 2011;39(1):134–9.
35. Redfern J, Kamath G, Burks R. Anatomical confirmation of the use of radiographic landmarks in medial patellofemoral ligament reconstruction. Am J Sports Med 2010;38(2):293–7.
36. Ostermeier S, Holst M, Hurschler C, et al. Dynamic measurement of patellofemoral kinematics and contact pressure after lateral retinacular release: an in vitro study. Knee Surg Sports Traumatol Arthrosc 2007;15(5):547–54.
37. Nonweiler DE, DeLee JC. The diagnosis and treatment of medial subluxation of the patella after lateral retinacular release. Am J Sports Med 1994;22(5):680–6.
38. Senavongse W, Amis AA. The effects of articular, retinacular, or muscular deficiencies on patellofemoral joint stability: a biomechanical study in vitro. J Bone Joint Surg Br 2005;87(4):577–82.
39. Senavongse W, Farahmand F, Jones J, et al. Quantitative measurement of patellofemoral joint stability: force-displacement behavior of the human patella in vitro. J Orthop Res 2003;21(5):780–6.
40. Smirk C, Morris H. The anatomy and reconstruction of the medial patellofemoral ligament. Knee 2003;10(3):221–7.
41. Beck P, Brown NA, Greis PE, et al. Patellofemoral contact pressures and lateral patellar translation after medial patellofemoral ligament reconstruction. Am J Sports Med 2007;35(9):1557–63.
42. Deie M, Ochi M, Sumen Y, et al. Reconstruction of the medial patellofemoral ligament for the treatment of habitual or recurrent dislocation of the patella in children. J Bone Joint Surg Br 2003;85(6):887–90.
43. Deie M, Ochi M, Sumen Y, et al. A long-term follow-up study after medial patellofemoral ligament reconstruction using the transferred semitendinosus tendon for patellar dislocation. Knee Surg Sports Traumatol Arthrosc 2005;13(7):522–8.
44. Ellera Gomes JL, Stigler Marczyk LR, César de César P, et al. Medial patellofemoral ligament reconstruction with semitendinosus autograft for chronic patellar instability: a follow-up study. Arthroscopy 2004;20(2):147–51.
45. Fernandez E, Sala D, Castejon M. Reconstruction of the medial patellofemoral ligament for patellar instability using a semitendinosus autograft. Acta Orthop Belg 2005;71(3):303–8.
46. Hinterwimmer S, Imhoff AB, Minzlaff P, et al. Anatomical two-bundle medial patellofemoral ligament reconstruction with hardware-free patellar graft fixation: technical note and preliminary results. Knee Surg Sports Traumatol Arthrosc 2013;21(9):2147–54.
47. Kohn LM, Meidinger G, Beitzel K, et al. Isolated and combined medial patellofemoral ligament reconstruction in revision surgery for patellofemoral instability: a prospective study. Am J Sports Med 2013;41(9):2128–35.
48. Mikashima Y, Kimura M, Kobayashi Y, et al. Clinical results of isolated reconstruction of the medial patellofemoral ligament for recurrent dislocation and subluxation of the patella. Acta Orthop Belg 2006;72(1):65–71.
49. Raghuveer RK, Mishra CB. Reconstruction of medial patellofemoral ligament for chronic patellar instability. Indian J Orthop 2012;46(4):447–54.

50. Schöttle PB, Fucentese SF, Romero J. Clinical and radiological outcome of medial patellofemoral ligament reconstruction with a semitendinosus autograft for patella instability. Knee Surg Sports Traumatol Arthrosc 2005;13(7):516–21.
51. Slenker NR, Tucker BS, Pepe MD, et al. Short-/intermediate-term outcomes after medial patellofemoral ligament reconstruction in the treatment of chronic lateral patellofemoral instability. Phys Sportsmed 2013;41(2):26–33.
52. Steiner TM, Torga-Spak R, Teitge RA. Medial patellofemoral ligament reconstruction in patients with lateral patellar instability and trochlear dysplasia. Am J Sports Med 2006;34(8):1254–61.
53. Thaunat M, Erasmus PJ. The favourable anisometry: an original concept for medial patellofemoral ligament reconstruction. Knee 2007;14(6):424–8.
54. Toritsuka Y, Amano H, Mae T, et al. Dual tunnel medial patellofemoral ligament reconstruction for patients with patellar dislocation using a semitendinosus tendon autograft. Knee 2011;18(4):214–9.
55. Watanabe T, Muneta T, Ikeda H, et al. Visual analog scale assessment after medial patellofemoral ligament reconstruction: with or without tibial tubercle transfer. J Orthop Sci 2008;13(1):32–8.

Distal Realignment
Indications, Technique, and Results

Kyle Duchman, MD*, Matt Bollier, MD

KEYWORDS

- Distal realignment • Patellar instability • Anterior knee pain
- Tibial tubercle osteotomy • Patellofemoral joint • Patellar tracking

KEY POINTS

- Distal realignment can be used with or without proximal stabilization in cases of patellofemoral instability when malalignment or a lateral tracking vector is present.
- Distal realignment is effective at unloading lateral and distal patellofemoral cartilage lesions.
- Anteromedialization allows for multiplanar adjustments while also providing a long, flat osteotomy that optimizes bone healing and screw placement.
- Distalization can be incorporated with anteromedialization to address patella alta.

INTRODUCTION

Distal realignment of the extensor mechanism can be used to address patellofemoral instability, to unload lateral or distal patella cartilage lesions, or to address lateral patella overload, tilt, and compression.

Stability of the patellofemoral joint relies on a complex interplay of bony anatomy, soft tissue restraints, and dynamic muscle action to maintain congruency of the joint. Multiple clinical and radiographic factors including ligamentous laxity, increased quadriceps angle (Q-angle), femoral anteversion, trochlear dysplasia, quadriceps dysplasia, excessive tibial tubercle-trochlear groove distance (TT-TG), and patella alta have been identified as risk factors for patellar instability and dislocation.[1–5]

More than 100 procedures have been described to address the various factors involved in patellar instability. Classically, acute patellar dislocations have been treated conservatively with a combination of early range of motion and quadriceps strengthening with or without bracing or taping.[6] Recurrent dislocation following conservative therapy occurs in 15% to 44% of patients, whereas a history of dislocation increases the risk of subsequent dislocation.[7,8] It is estimated that upwards of 50% of dislocations occur during sports, with football and basketball the most frequently cited

Department of Orthopaedics and Rehabilitation, University of Iowa Hospitals and Clinics, 200 Hawkins Drive, 01008 JPP, Iowa City, IA 52242, USA
* Corresponding author.
E-mail address: kyle-duchman@uiowa.edu

Clin Sports Med 33 (2014) 517–530
http://dx.doi.org/10.1016/j.csm.2014.03.001
0278-5919/14/$ – see front matter © 2014 Elsevier Inc. All rights reserved.
sportsmed.theclinics.com

activity at the time of injury.[6,7,9,10] Anatomically, disruption of the medial patellofe-moral ligament (MPFL), the primary soft tissue restraint to lateral patellar translation, has been identified as the essential lesion following acute patellar dislocation. MPFL reconstruction has become a popular option to address patellofemoral instability and is indicated in cases of recurrent instability with a normal tracking vector and defi-cient proximal soft tissue restraints. However, isolated MPFL reconstruction fails to address patella alta or extensor mechanism malalignment. Now more than a century old, distal realignment procedures, including the tibial tubercle osteotomy, aim to cor-rect the orientation of the extensor mechanism. The original tibial tubercle osteotomy medialized the distal extensor mechanism, aiming to correct the clinical Q-angle and radiographic TT-TG distance.

Modifications of the original description have since been developed to allow multi-planar correction of the distal extensor mechanism. Several authors also describe distal realignment procedures to unload cartilage lesions of the patella.[11,12] Precise cuts allow adjustments to be made in the axial, coronal, and sagittal planes with the ability to tailor treatment to an individual patient's pathology. Anteromedialization of the tibial tubercle was first described by Fulkerson in 1983.[13] This method allowed the obliquity of the osteotomy to be adjusted to provide more medialization, to address lateral instability, or more anteriorization, to unload lateral and distal patella cartilage lesions. In addition, the long, flat osteotomy created during anteromedializa-tion provided increased surface area to enhance healing while also providing a large bone block to accommodate screw placement. In addition, tibial tubercle osteotomies have been combined with other soft tissue and bony procedures, including MPFL reconstruction, lateral retinacular release, and trochleoplasty, to individualize therapy even further. As the trend toward individualized treatment continues, understanding the subtleties of patellofemoral pathology and the effect a specific surgical interven-tion has on that pathology becomes essential for the treating surgeon in order to opti-mize outcomes.

This review aims to provide an overview of distal realignment procedures while focusing on the indications for surgery and surgical technique. In providing this infor-mation, anatomic and biomechanical considerations that affect surgical planning and decision-making are discussed. In addition, current issues and controversies related to distal realignment procedures are discussed throughout the review.

INDICATIONS

Indications for distal realignment are variable throughout the literature, but the most frequently cited indications include lateral patellofemoral instability, anterior knee pain with associated lateral or distal patellofemoral cartilage lesions, and lateral patellar overload or tilt. Careful patient selection is critical for successful outcomes following distal realignment procedures.

When patients with patellofemoral instability fail to respond to nonoperative man-agement, it can be difficult to determine the most appropriate surgical technique to address instability. It is important to determine first whether proximal stabilization, distal realignment, or both, is needed (**Fig. 1**).

In cases of recurrent patellofemoral instability, confirmation of the diagnosis and ex-amination for risk factors (trochlear dysplasia, patella alta, hyperlaxity, and malalign-ment) are the first steps.[3] The moving patella apprehension test dynamically stresses the patella during physiologic knee range of motion to determine the ade-quacy of the MPFL, as it serves to pull the patella into the trochlear groove during knee flexion.[14] The vector of the quadriceps, frequently referred to as the "Q-angle,"

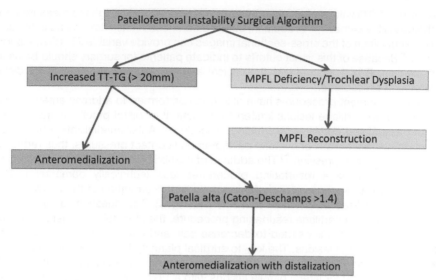

Fig. 1. A patellofemoral instability treatment algorithm.

can also be assessed clinically and is defined as the angle created by the resultant vector of the quadriceps as it passes through the center of the patella and the tibial tubercle.[15] Although a pathologic threshold has yet to be established, normal Q-angle values are reported between 14 and 23°.[16,17] As the value of the Q-angle increases, the resultant lateral force on the patella also increases, contributing to lateral patellar translation.[18] Unfortunately, much variability within populations as well as poor correlation to more reliable radiographic measures, such as the TT-TG distance,[19] has called into question the utility of the Q-angle measurement for preoperative assessment.

Initial radiographic imaging during the evaluation of the patient with patellar instability should consist of standing anteroposterior and lateral views of the knee as well as axial tangential views of the patellofemoral joint, such as the Merchant view.[20] These standard radiographs allow for evaluation of the severity and location of patellofemoral osteoarthritis, both of which have been shown to affect subjective outcomes after distal realignment procedures.[21,22] These views also allow for assessment of patellar height, with Caton-Deschamps and Insall-Salvati indices greater than 1.2 suggested as a consideration for distalization of the tibial tubercle during distal realignment procedures.[23,24] The authors typically perform distalization of the osteotomized tubercle with a Caton-Deschamps index greater than 1.4. Dejour and colleagues[3] defined 4 radiographic risk factors for instability, including (1) trochlear dysplasia, which was referred to as the "fundamental factor" of instability; (2) quadriceps dysplasia, expressed radiographically as patellar tilt; (3) patella alta, defined as a Caton-Deschamps[25] index greater than 1.2; and (4) TT-TG distance greater than 20 mm.[3] The TT-TG distance is measured by taking a line perpendicular to a line tangential to the posterior femoral condyles through the deepest part of the trochlear groove and through the apex of the tibial tubercle, again perpendicular to the line tangential to the posterior femoral condyles. The distance between these 2 lines is defined as the TT-TG distance. Although originally described for computed tomography (CT), other cross-sectional imaging modalities, such as magnetic resonance imaging (MRI), have been used to calculate the TT-TG distance. Although these modalities may allow better visualization of soft tissue structures involved in patellar instability, TT-TG values often differ between CT and MRI, although the measurement technique is the same.[26,27] In addition, subtle differences in knee flexion and extension during acquisition of the cross-sectional images can provide variable TT-TG measurements.[28] Because of this, strict cutoffs to indicate patients for surgery should be used with caution. **Box 1** summarizes the clinical and radiographic indications for distal realignment procedures.

Distal realignment procedures have also been performed to address anterior knee pain related to cartilage lesions limited to the lateral or distal patella facets with or without associated cartilage resurfacing procedures. Anteromedialization has been shown to decrease distal and lateral patellofemoral contact pressures, thus reducing lateral trochlear compression.[29] The addition of the tibial tubercle osteotomy can also make patella cartilage resurfacing procedures less technically demanding. The osteotomy allows easier eversion of the patella and visualization of the cartilaginous defect, as visualized in the case presented in **Fig. 2**. The question remains as to whether the patella cartilage resurfacing procedure, the tibial tubercle osteotomy, or a combination of both is needed to decrease pain and improve function in patients with patella cartilage lesions. The key to surgical planning is to know the location of the lesion and the TT-TG distance. The authors recommend an isolated anteromedialization osteotomy for lateral patella lesions with a TT-TG greater than 15 mm. If the TT-TG is less than 10 mm, the osteotomy should be oriented to shift only the tubercle anteriorly. When the TT-TG is corrected to less than 12 mm and there is no residual instability, results of cell-based resurfacing procedures have shown favorable results.[30]

Because of the multitude of factors that can produce anterior knee pain, distinguishing the exact source of anterior knee pain can be difficult, even after a meticulous history and physical examination.[4] Multiple anatomic sources including the synovium, subchondral bone, retinaculum, skin, muscle, and nerve can serve as pain generators for patients presenting with anterior knee pain.[4] Furthermore, positive outcomes following distal realignment procedures for patients with anterior knee pain as an isolated complaint are less reproducible than for patients with objective patellar instability.[22] Thus, surgery is indicated for anterior knee pain only when a specific anatomic factor, such as a cartilage lesion, can be addressed.

Contraindications

There are relatively few absolute contraindications for distal realignment procedures. Most would agree that all efforts should be made to delay surgery until the closure of

---

Box 1
Indications for distal realignment procedures

1. Recurrent patellofemoral instability in patients with:
   - Skeletal maturity (closed physes)
   - TT-TG >15–20 mm
   - Caton-Deschamps >1.4
2. Unload focal patella cartilage lesion
   - Without cartilage resurfacing for lateral or distal lesions
   - With cartilage resurfacing for central or medial lesion
3. Isolated lateral patellofemoral compression, tilt, or overload in patients who fail an attempt at lateral release

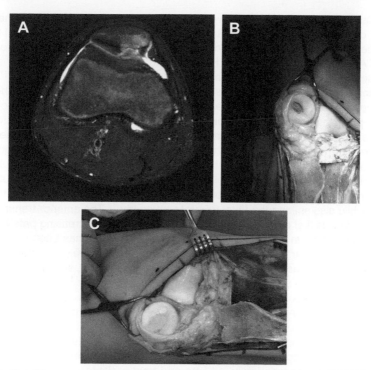

Fig. 2. (*A–C*) A 21-year-old woman with a history of patellofemoral instability and a large, symptomatic patella cartilage lesion. Her TT-TG distance measured 21 mm preoperatively without evidence of patella alta. An anteromedial tibial tubercle transfer was performed to unload the symptomatic cartilage lesion in addition to cartilage resurfacing. (*A*) Preoperative T2-weighted MRI reveals a large patella cartilage lesion without evidence of a trochlear lesion. (*B*) Intraoperative image confirms large, central cartilaginous defect with patella everted following osteotomy of the tibial tubercle. (*C*) Everted image of the cartilaginous patella lesion after resurfacing and before definitive fixation of the osteotomized tubercle.

the proximal tibial physis and apophysis of the tibial tubercle,[31,32] related to reports of genu recurvatum in patients under 14 years of age undergoing distal realignment procedures.[33,34] Given that the average age of index dislocation in patients occurs between 14 and 17 years,[6,7,9,10] surgery can typically be delayed with conservative management and activity modification if needed until physeal closure.

Relative contraindications to medial tibial tubercle transfer also include a history of medial patellar dislocation or subluxation, because further medialization of the distal extensor mechanism may increase the risk for subsequent medial dislocation events.[35] In addition, the relatively poor outcomes in patients who present with diffuse patellofemoral arthrosis makes distal realignment procedures a poor choice in this population.[21,22,36] Isolated medialization is typically avoided in cases where there are cartilage lesions of the medial patella or trochlea, but transfer in other planes may still be performed.[37]

SURGICAL TECHNIQUE
History of Distal Realignment Procedures

The first description of a distal realignment procedure was provided by Roux[38] in 1888 to address recurrent patellar dislocation. The Roux procedure included medial retinacular plication and lateral release in addition to a medial transfer of the lateral one-half of the patellar tendon by rotating the released portion of the lateral patellar tendon behind the medial patellar tendon with suture fixation to the proximal tibial periosteum. At nearly the same time as Roux, Goldthwait[39] described a similar surgical technique, thus popularizing the Roux-Goldthwait procedure.

Modifications of Roux's original description have subsequently been published. Trillat and colleagues[40] described the technique first used by Elmslie, which included a flat axial plane osteotomy of the tibial tubercle with medial transfer, now popularly known as the Elmslie-Trillat procedure. Hauser,[41] in an attempt to correct the patella alta he frequently saw associated with recurrent patellar dislocation, described a tibial tubercle osteotomy with distal translation of the osteotomy. More recently, multiplanar osteotomies, such as the oblique tibial tubercle osteotomy described by Fulkerson, allow correction of the distal extensor mechanism through medialization of the tibial tubercle while also shifting the tibial tubercle anteriorly.[42] The anterior transfer of the tibial tubercle was first described by Maquet[43] in hopes of decreasing patellofemoral joint forces and pain in patients with instability. This practice has been incorporated into several multiplanar techniques. Biomechanical models have suggested that anteromedialization decreases pressure on the lateral patellar facet, which may serve as a source of knee pain in some individuals with patellar instability.[12] Multiplanar osteotomies allow surgeons to tailor treatment of individuals with variable risk factors, including increased Q-angle, increased TT-TG distance, or patella alta, that may simultaneously contribute to an individual's patellar instability. The ability of each procedure to correct specific anatomic factors related to patellar instability makes it essential that the orthopedic surgeon understand the complex pathophysiology of patellar instability to appropriately indicate and treat patients.

Medialization of the Tibial Tubercle

Isolated medialization of the tibial tubercle was the first described distal realignment procedure.[38] Medialization of the tibial tubercle decreases the resultant lateral force vector acting on the patella by medializing the most distal aspect of the extensor mechanism. In doing so, the pressure on the patellar articular cartilage, primarily the lateral facet, can be reduced significantly.[12,44,45] The desired amount of medialization varies throughout the literature, with postoperative TT-TG goals ranging from 9 to 15 mm.[24,46–49] When assessing the adequacy of medialization intraoperatively with passive or active range of motion, the amount of medialization required to prevent subluxation is increased in patients who present with instability as opposed to pain.[22] The amount of isolated medialization that can be achieved is limited by the amount of bony contact available between the osteotomized tubercle and tibia because of the triangular shape of the tibia. Medialization has produced good clinical results, with low rates of postoperative dislocation and improved subjective outcome scores.[31,50] However, there is concern that pain and patellofemoral arthrosis may occur at an increased rate at long-term follow-up after isolated medialization.[51]

Distalization of the Tibial Tubercle

Isolated distalization of the tibial tubercle is rarely indicated because patella alta typically occurs in conjunction with other instability factors, and therefore, a multiplanar osteotomy is more commonly described. Indications for distalization include Caton-Deschamps or Insall-Salvati indices greater than 1.2.[23,24] The authors typically elect to perform distalization as a component of the multiplanar osteotomy when the Caton-Deschamps index measures greater than 1.4 mm, as demonstrated in **Fig. 3**. Care must be taken to avoid overdistalization, which may limit knee flexion.

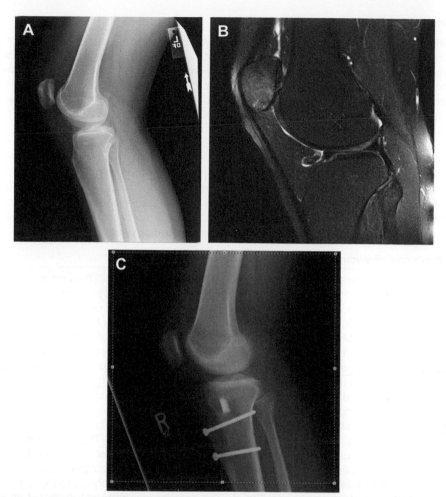

Fig. 3. (*A–C*) A 20-year-old woman with a history of recurrent patellofemoral instability with an intra-articular loose body originating from the patella. Her preoperative TT-TG and Caton-Deschamps measurements were 19 mm and 1.4, respectively. (*A*) Preoperative lateral radiograph demonstrating Caton-Deschamps index measured greater than 1.4, the authors preferred cutoff for distalization. (*B*) Preoperative sagittal T2-weighted MRI reveals an intra-articular loose body. (*C*) A postoperative lateral radiograph after anteromedialization and combined distalization of the tibial tubercle shows correction of the Caton-Deschamps index.

Anteriorization of the Tibial Tubercle

Originally described by Maquet,[43] isolated anterior transfer was first performed for chondromalacia patellae in hopes of reducing patellofemoral contact pressures and pain. There were significant issues with fixation, because an autograft or allograft bone block was needed to achieve fixation. Because of these issues, isolated anteriorization of the tibial tubercle is not commonly used. However, Rue and colleagues[37] reported that pure anteriorization may be advantageous in patients with medial articular cartilage lesions for which anteromedialization is contraindicated. Anteriorization is still a vital component of the multiplanar anteromedialization procedure popularized by Fulkerson and described in later discussion.[42]

Anteromedialization of the Tibial Tubercle

Originally described by Fulkerson in 1983, anteromedialization of the tibial tubercle aims to combine the positive effects of isolated medial and anterior tibial tubercle transfer while addressing the shortcoming of each isolated procedure, namely, the requirement for bone graft and limited surface area for healing of the osteotomy, respectively.[13] The Fulkerson anteromedialization osteotomy provides several advantages. First, the long, flat osteotomy provides a large cancellous surface area to enhance bone healing and provides adequate area to place several screws. Second, the distal taper as the osteotomy nears the tibial crest reduces the risk of a tibia fracture. Last, the angle of the oblique axial plane osteotomy can be adjusted to accommodate the pathologic condition for a specific patient, allowing for various amounts of anterior and medial translation to be achieved. In addition, anteromedialization has been shown to reduce contact pressure on the patellar cartilage while also correcting patellar maltracking in biomechanical models.[45] **Box 2** summarizes the advantages and disadvantages of the Fulkerson or anteromedialization procedure.

Anteromedialization: A Detailed Surgical Technique

The patient is placed in the supine position with a tourniquet positioned on the proximal thigh of the operative extremity. The lower extremity is prepared from the thigh to the foot using a chlorhexidine-based solution. Draping is carried out in the standard sterile fashion to allow full knee range of motion for the operative lower extremity.

The procedure begins with a diagnostic arthroscopy of the affected knee using standard anteromedial and lateral portals. The severity and location of cartilage damage should be noted as should the tracking of the patella with passive knee range of motion. If indicated preoperatively, arthroscopic lateral release or medial plication can also be performed at this time. A tourniquet is used throughout the duration of the case until assessing hemostasis before wound closure.

After diagnostic arthroscopy, attention is turned toward the tibial tubercle. An incision measuring 5 to 6 cm is made just lateral to the tibial tubercle. The incision should be made large enough to limit damage to the skin and soft tissues during creation of the osteotomy. Dissection is continued sharply to the level of the patella tendon insertion on the tibial tubercle, and a hemostat is placed behind the tendon to free it from the underlying metaphyseal bone (**Fig. 4**). The anterior compartment musculature is then elevated from the lateral edge of the tibial crest and retracted posteriorly to expose the posterior aspect of the tibia. Retractors are then placed to expose the entire length of the planned osteotomy.

The amount of medialization and anteriorization is determined by the obliquity of the osteotomy in the axial plane, with a more oblique (anterior to posterior) osteotomy producing more anteriorization for unloading of lateral and distal cartilaginous lesions.

Box 2
Advantages and disadvantages of anteromedialization/Fulkerson procedure

Advantages	Disadvantages
Preservation of the extensor mechanism	Fails to address incompetent MPFL
Large surface area for bone healing	Postoperative hardware irritation
Ability to place multiple screws	Potential neurovascular injury
Multiplanar adjustments	Increased medial patellofemoral contact pressure
Early range of motion	Delayed union or nonunion
	Cannot be performed in skeletally immature

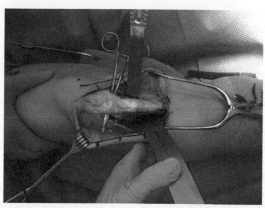

Fig. 4. An intraoperative photograph shows the exposed tibial tubercle before performing the oblique osteotomy. Note the snap placed under the most distal aspect of the patella tendon as it inserts on the tuberosity.

After adequate exposure of the lateral surface of the tibia, electrocautery is used to mark the planned osteotomy. The osteotomy line is drawn to merge with the anterior tibial cortex at the most distal aspect of the osteotomy. Several guides exist to aid in creation of the osteotomy, but the senior author's preferred technique is a free-hand technique. The osteotomy cut is created using an oscillating saw from medial to lateral and anterior to posterior along the oblique axial plane. The cut should begin at the most distal aspect of the planned osteotomy and proceed proximally. An attempt should be made to leave a distal periosteal hinge along the tibial crest unless concomitant distalization is indicated. Avoiding damage to the surrounding soft tissues is critical during this step. The oblique osteotomy is completed with an osteotome. A 0.25-inch osteotome is used from lateral to medial just proximal to the patella tendon insertion on the tubercle to create a proximal bumper. The final cut to mobilize the tibial tubercle bone block is made using a 0.5-inch osteotome to connect the oblique osteotomy to the proximal bumper.

At this point, the osteotomized tubercle can be rotated anteriorly and medially along the oblique plane of the osteotomy. Temporary fixation of the tibial tubercle can be achieved using two 0.062-inch Kirschner wires to allow intraoperative assessment of patellar tracking. Assessment of the patellofemoral joint can be achieved by passively taking the knee through a full range of motion. Assessment of the patella after provisional fixation can also be achieved arthroscopically to visualize tracking. Special attention should be made to avoid overmedialization of extensor mechanism resulting in medial tracking. Typically, medialization greater than 1 cm is not recommended.

Definitive fixation of the osteotomized fragment is achieved using 4.5-mm self-tapping screws using a lag technique by overdrilling the near cortex. Screw placement is approximately 1 cm distal to the patella tendon insertion and screws are spaced 2 cm apart to reduce the risk of fracture. The screws should be aimed as perpendicular as possible to the osteotomy plane. Biomechanical testing has shown increased load to failure with two 4.5-mm screws as opposed to three 3.5-mm screws, although this difference was not statistically significant.[52] After the osteotomized tubercle is secured, attention can be turned to proximal stabilization procedures as indicated.

At this point the tourniquet is taken down and hemostasis is achieved. A final diagnostic arthroscopic examination can be performed at this time to assess patella tracking. Fine adjustments in tracking can be made by restoring or releasing retinaculum arthroscopically.

COMPLICATIONS

Overall complications following distal realignment procedures have been reported at 7.4%.[47] The most frequently reported complication following distal realignment procedures is symptomatic hardware, with as many as 50% of patients requiring subsequent hardware removal for hardware irritation.[49,53] In addition, superficial surgical site infections and deep venous thrombosis have been reported, both of which are most frequently medically managed and resolve appropriately. More concerning complications, including fractures of the proximal tibia, have been reported at low rates ranging from 1% to 2.6%.[47,54] These fractures typically heal with cast immobilization for 6 to 8 weeks with open reduction internal fixation rarely required.[22,36,47,54] Other less frequently reported complications include painful neuroma, arthrofibrosis, nonunion of the osteotomized tubercle, anterior tibial artery or deep peroneal nerve injury, osteomyelitis, and medial patellar dislocation.[23,24]

POSTOPERATIVE MANAGEMENT

Patients should remain non-weight-bearing on the operative extremity with the use of crutches for 6 weeks postoperatively. However, early range of motion, starting as early as postoperative day 1, is recommended to prevent flexion contractures postoperatively. More conservative weight-bearing measures are used because immediate weight-bearing resulted in a relatively high incidence of proximal tibial fractures compared with non-weight-bearing protocols.[54] While ambulating, the knee should remain in extension through the use of either a knee immobilizer or a hinged knee brace locked in extension. Formal physical therapy for any loss of motion and quadriceps strengthening should be started 6 weeks postoperatively. Most patients discontinue crutches by 8 weeks postoperatively.

OUTCOMES

Comparison of outcomes following distal realignment procedures is difficult given that several indications for distal realignment exist and often is performed as a combined procedure with proximal stabilization procedures. In addition, "distal realignment procedure" is a generic term for several specific procedures, each with a slightly different role in the treatment of patellar instability or patellofemoral pain and is emphasized by the fact that the only meta-analysis available on nonoperative versus operative management of patellar dislocation includes a single nonrandomized control study that used distal realignment.[55]

Distal realignment procedures do provide good results when appropriately indicated. Rates of dislocation following surgery are low with the rate of dislocation varying from 0% to 15.2%.[10,31,48,49,53,56] Interpretation of these results should be made with caution, because persistent subjective instability and frank postoperative dislocation are often grouped together in the literature. Tjoumakaris and colleagues[53] recently reported on 41 Fulkerson osteotomies in 34 athletes who presented for patellofemoral instability. They reportedly significant improvement in both Lysholm and International Knee Documentation Committee (IKDC) scores at a mean follow-up of 46 months. In their study, only one recurrent dislocation was noted, while hardware removal was necessary in 49% of patients.

Subjectively, good or excellent results have been reported in 63% to 90% of patients following distal realignment procedures.[10,21–23,36,57] Persistent patellofemoral pain is one of the most frequently reported complaints postoperatively and is most likely to progress in studies providing long-term follow-up beyond 45 months.[51] Positive prognostic factors include male sex, grade 1 or 2 cartilage lesions as compared with grades 3 or 4 lesions, and instability predominant symptoms.[22,36] Distal realignment procedures do alter patellofemoral contact pressures and continued radiographic progression of arthrosis is frequently reported, which may contribute to deterioration of clinical results at longer follow-up.[51,56,58]

SUMMARY

When appropriately indicated, distal realignment procedures can produce consistent clinical results. Indications for distal realignment include lateral patellofemoral instability, anterior knee pain with associated lateral or distal patellofemoral cartilage lesion, and cases with significant lateral patellofemoral overload or tilt. In cases of patellofemoral instability, it is important to determine whether proximal stabilization, distal realignment, or both is needed. If distal realignment is indicated, several anatomic variables must be considered to determine the location and obliquity of the osteotomy when using multiplanar osteotomy techniques.

REFERENCES

1. Balcarek P, Jung K, Frosch KH, et al. Value of the tibial tuberosity-trochlear groove distance in patellar instability in the young athlete. Am J Sports Med 2011;39(8):1756–61.
2. Colvin AC, West RV. Patellar instability. J Bone Joint Surg Am 2008;90(12):12.
3. Dejour H, Walch G, Nove-Josserand L, et al. Factors of patellar instability: an anatomic radiographic study. Knee Surg Sports Traumatol Arthrosc 1994;2:8.
4. Fulkerson JP. Diagnosis and treatment of patients with patellofemoral pain. Am J Sports Med 2002;30(3):10.
5. Redziniak DE, Diduch DR, Mihalko WM, et al. Patellar instability. J Bone Joint Surg Am 2009;91(9):12.
6. Garth WP, Pomphrey M, Merrill K. Functional treatment of patellar dislocation in an athletic population. Am J Sports Med 1996;24(6):7.
7. Fithian DC, Paxton EW, Stone ML, et al. Epidemiology and natural history of acute patellar dislocation. Am J Sports Med 2004;32(5):1114–21.
8. Hawkins RJ, Bell RH, Anisette G. Acute patellar dislocations: the natural history. Am J Sports Med 1986;32:8.
9. Lewallen LW, McIntosh AL, Dahm DL. Predictors of recurrent instability after acute patellofemoral dislocation in pediatric and adolescent patients. Am J Sports Med 2013;41(3):575–81.
10. Garth WP, DiChristina DG, Holt G. Delayed proximal repair and distal realignment after patellar dislocation. Clin Orthop Relat Res 2000;(377):132–44.
11. Saleh KJ, Arendt EA, Eldridge J, et al. Operative treatment of patellofemoral arthritis. J Bone Joint Surg Am 2005;87:13.
12. Saranathan A, Kirkpatrick MS, Mani S, et al. The effect of tibial tuberosity realignment procedures on the patellofemoral pressure distribution. Knee Surg Sports Traumatol Arthrosc 2012;20(10):2054–61.
13. Fulkerson JP. Anteromedialization of the tibial tuberosity for patellofemoral malalignment. Clin Orthop Relat Res 1983;(177):176–81.

14. Ahmad CS, McCarthy M, Gomez JA, et al. The moving patellar apprehension test for lateral patellar instability. Am J Sports Med 2009;37(4):6.
15. Brattstrom H. Patella alta in non-dislocating knee joints. Acta Orthop Scand 1970;41(5):11.
16. Fairbank J, Pynsent PB, van Poortvliet JA, et al. Mechanical factors in the incidence of knee pain in adolescents and young adults. J Bone Joint Surg Br 1984; 66(5):9.
17. Insall J, Falvo KA, Wise DW. Chondromalacia patellae: a prospective study. J Bone Joint Surg Am 1976;58(1):1–8.
18. Bicos J, Carofino B, Andersen M, et al. Patellofemoral forces after medial patellofemoral ligament reconstruction: a biomechanical analysis. J Knee Surg 2006; 19(4):10.
19. Cooney AD, Kazi Z, Caplan N, et al. The relationship between quadriceps angle and tibial tuberosity-trochlear groove distance in patients with patellar instability. Knee Surg Sports Traumatol Arthrosc 2012;20(12):2399–404.
20. Merchant AC, Mercer RL, Jacobsen RH, et al. Roentgenographic analysis of patellofemoral congruence. J Bone Joint Surg Am 1974;56:6.
21. Pidoriano AJ, Weinstein RN, Buuck DA, et al. Correlation of patellar articular lesions with results from anteromedial tibial tubercle transfer. Am J Sports Med 1997;25(4):5.
22. Pritsch T, Haim A, Arbel R, et al. Tailored tibial tubercle transfer for patellofemoral malalignment: analysis of clinical outcomes. Knee Surg Sports Traumatol Arthrosc 2007;15(8):994–1002.
23. Cootjans K, Dujardin J, Vandenneucker H, et al. A surgical algorithm for the treatment of recurrent patellar dislocation. Results at 5 year follow-up. Acta Orthop Belg 2013;79:318–25.
24. Feller JA. Distal realignment (tibial tuberosity transfer). Sports Med Arthrosc Rev 2012;20:10.
25. Caton J, Deschamps G, Chambat P, et al. Patella Infera. Apropos of 128 cases. Rev Chir Orthop Reparatrice Appar Mot 1982;68(5):317–25.
26. Camp CL, Stuart MJ, Krych AJ, et al. CT and MRI measurements of tibial tubercle-trochlear groove distances are not equivalent in patients with patellar instability. Am J Sports Med 2013;41(8):1835–40.
27. Schoettle PB, Zanetti M, Seifert B, et al. The tibial tuberosity-trochlear groove distance; a comparative study between CT and MRI scanning. Knee 2006;13(1):26–31.
28. Dietrich TJ, Betz M, Pfirrmann CW, et al. End-stage extension of the knee and its influence on tibial tuberosity-trochlear groove distance (TTTG) in asymptomatic volunteers. Knee Surg Sports Traumatol Arthrosc 2014;22(1):214–8.
29. Beck PR, Thomas AL, Farr J, et al. Trochlear contact pressures are anteromedialization of the tibial tubercle. Am J Sports Med 2005;33(11):6.
30. Peterson L, Brittberg M, Kiviranta I, et al. Autologous chondrocyte implantation. Biomechanics and long-term durability. Am J Sports Med 2002;30(1):11.
31. Barber FA, McGarry JE. Elmslie-Trillat procedure for the treatment of recurrent patellar instability. Arthroscopy 2008;24(1):77–81.
32. Hinton RY, Sharma KM. Acute and recurrent patellar instability in the young athlete. Orthop Clin North Am 2003;34(3):385–96.
33. Harrison MH. The results of a realignment operation for recurrent dislocation of the patella. J Bone Joint Surg Br 1955;37(4):559–67.
34. Macnab I. Recurrent dislocation of the patella. J Bone Joint Surg Am 1952;34(4):11.
35. Bicos J, Fulkerson JP. Indications and technique of distal tibial tubercle anteromedialization. Operat Tech Orthop 2007;17(4):223–33.

36. Wang CJ, Chan YS, Chen HH, et al. Factors affecting the outcome of distal realignment for patellofemoral disorders of the knee. Knee 2005;12(3): 195–200.
37. Rue JP, Colton A, Zare SM, et al. Trochlear contact pressures after straight anteriorization of the tibial tuberosity. Am J Sports Med 2008;36(10):7.
38. Roux C. Luxation habituelle de la rotule: traitement operatoire. Rev Chir Orthop Reparatrice Appar Mot 1888;8:8.
39. Goldthwait JE. Permanent dislocation of the patella. The report of a case of twenty years' duration, successfully treated by transplantation of the patella tendons with the tubercle of the tibia. Ann Surg 1899;29(1):62–8.
40. Trillat A, Dejour H, Couette A. Diagnosis and treatment of recurrent dislocations of the patella. Rev Chir Orthop Reparatrice Appar Mot 1964;50:12.
41. Hauser EW. Total tendon transplant for slipping patella. Surg Gynecol Obstet 1938;66:16.
42. Fulkerson JP, Becker GJ, Meaney JA, et al. Anteromedial tibial tubercle transfer without bone graft. Am J Sports Med 1990;18(5):7.
43. Maquet P. Compression strain in the patello-femoral joint. Acta Orthop Belg 1981;47(1):5.
44. Kuroda R, Kambic H, Vealdevit A, et al. Articular cartilage contact pressure after tibial tuberosity transfer: a cadaveric study. Am J Sports Med 2001;29(4):7.
45. Ramappa AJ, Apreleva M, Harrold FR, et al. The effects of medialization and anteromedialization of the tibial tubercle on patellofemoral mechanics and kinematics. Am J Sports Med 2006;34(5):749–56.
46. Dejour D, Le Coultre B. Osteotomies in patello-femoral instabilities. Sports Med Arthrosc Rev 2007;15:8.
47. Servien E, Verdonk PC, Neyret P. Tibial tuberosity transfer for episodic patellar dislocation. Sports Med Arthrosc Rev 2007;15(2):7.
48. Tecklenburg K, Feller JA, Whitehead TS, et al. Outcome of surgery for recurrent patellar dislocation based on the distance of the tibial tuberosity to the trochlear groove. J Bone Joint Surg Br 2010;92:5.
49. Koeter S, Diks MJ, Anderson PG, et al. A modified tibial tubercle osteotomy for patellar maltracking: results at two years. J Bone Joint Surg Br 2007;89:6.
50. Carney JR, Mologne TS, Muldoon M, et al. Long-term evaluation of the Roux-Elmslie-Trillat procedure for patellar instability: a 26-year follow-up. Am J Sports Med 2005;33(8):4.
51. Nakagawa K, Wada Y, Minamide M, et al. Deterioration of long-term clinical results after Elmslie-Trillat procedure for dislocation of the patella. J Bone Joint Surg Br 2002;84:4.
52. Warner BT, Kamath GV, Spang JT, et al. Comparison of fixation methods after anteromedialization osteotomy of the tibial tubercle for patellar instability. Arthroscopy 2013;29(10):1628–34.
53. Tjoumakaris FP, Forsythe B, Bradley JP. Patellofemoral instability in athletes: treatment via modified Fulkerson osteotomy and lateral release. Am J Sports Med 2010;38(5):992–9.
54. Stetson WB, Friedman MJ, Fulkerson JP, et al. Fracture of the proximal tibia with immediate weightbearing after a Fulkerson osteotomy. Am J Sports Med 1997;25(4):5.
55. Smith TO, Song F, Donell ST, et al. Operative versus non-operative management of patellar dislocation. A meta-analysis. Knee Surg Sports Traumatol Arthrosc 2011;19(6):988–98.
56. Sillanpaa P, Mattila VM, Visuri T, et al. Ligament reconstruction versus distal realignment for patellar dislocation. Clin Orthop Relat Res 2008;466(6):1475–84.

57. Henderson I, Francisco R. Treatment outcome of extensor realignment for patellofemoral dysfunction. Knee 2005;12(4):323–8.
58. Arnbjornsson A, Egund N, Rydling O, et al. The natural history of recurrent dislocation of the patella. Long-term results of conservative and operative treatment. J Bone Joint Surg Br 1992;74:3.

Trochlear Dysplasia and the Role of Trochleoplasty

Robert F. LaPrade, MD, PhD[a,b,]*, Tyler R. Cram, MA, ATC, OTC[a],
Evan W. James, BS[b], Matthew T. Rasmussen, BS[c]

KEYWORDS

• Patellar instability • Trochleoplasty • Trochlear dysplasia • Patellofemoral joint

KEY POINTS

• Patients with trochlear dysplasia frequently have recurrent patellar instability.
• Imaging is the most useful diagnostic technique for classifying trochlear morphology, assessing the severity of dysplasia, and assisting in preoperative planning.
• In many patients, a trochleoplasty permanently restores bony patellofemoral joint stability.
• A trochleoplasty is often performed alongside other patellar reconstruction procedures, including a medial patellofemoral ligament reconstruction or a tibial tubercle osteotomy.
• Patients with open physes or with advanced patellofemoral arthritis should not be considered candidates for a trochleoplasty.

INTRODUCTION

The incidence of primary patellar dislocation is estimated at 5.8 cases per 100,000 individuals.[1] In the at-risk population, which includes patients from 10 to 17 years of age, the incidence of patellar dislocation increases to 29 cases per 100,000 individuals. Recurrent dislocations reportedly occur in 17% of all cases following a primary dislocation event. After a second dislocation, the chance of additional dislocations increases to approximately 50%. For this reason, treatment is imperative for patients

Conflict of interest: The authors report no conflicts regarding board member/owner/officer/committee appointments, royalties, speaker's bureau/paid presentations, unpaid consultantships, research or institutional support from publishers, or stock or stock options. R.F. LaPrade is a paid consultant for Arthrex and receives research or institutional support from the Steadman Philippon Research Institute, which receives financial support from Smith & Nephew Endoscopy; Arthrex, Inc; Siemens Medical Solutions, USA; Sonoma Orthopedics, Inc; ConMed Linvatec; Össur Americas; Small Bone Innovations, Inc; Opedix; and Evidence Based Apparel.
a The Steadman Clinic, 181 West Meadow Drive, Suite 400, Vail, CO 81657, USA; b Center for Outcomes-based Orthopaedic Research, Steadman Philippon Research Institute, 181 West Meadow Drive, Suite 1000, Vail, CO 81657, USA; c Department of BioMedical Engineering, Steadman, Philippon Research Institute, 181 West Meadow Drive, Suite 1000, Vail, CO 81657, USA
* Corresponding author. The Steadman Clinic, 181 West Meadow Drive, Suite 400, Vail, CO 81657.
E-mail address: drlaprade@sprivail.org

who experience recurrent patellofemoral dislocations because symptoms often do not spontaneously resolve.

Chronic patellar instability is thought to have a multifactorial cause. In a normal patellofemoral joint, the combination of osseous stabilizers in the trochlea and medial soft tissue static stabilizers such as the medial patellofemoral ligament function to resist lateral patellar translation and to maintain patellofemoral stability. Patients with chronic instability routinely present with risk factors for recurrent dislocations, including trochlear dysplasia, patella alta, an increased tibial tubercle–trochlear groove (TT-TG) distance, and insufficiencies in the medial retinacular structures.[2]

Trochlear dysplasia is reportedly present in 85% of patients with patellar instability.[3] For patients with chronic instability secondary to trochlear dysplasia, the trochleoplasty procedure can be an effective treatment option to permanently restore stability.[4] This article highlights the basic anatomy and biomechanics of the patellofemoral joint, describes diagnostic imaging techniques to define and classify trochlear dysplasia, presents indications and the surgical technique for a sulcus-deepening trochleoplasty, and summarizes postsurgical outcomes.

NORMAL TROCHLEAR ANATOMY AND BIOMECHANICS
Anatomy

Normal trochlear bony anatomy confers many biomechanical advantages that contribute to patellofemoral joint stability. The trochlea is located on the anterodistal end of the femur and comprises medial and lateral facets and a central trochlear groove. The lateral facet is the larger of the two facets and extends further proximally.[5,6] The trochlear groove courses through the middle of the trochlea and divides the medial and lateral facets.[5,7] The trochlear groove deepens as it courses distally and its alignment deviates laterally with respect to the anatomic axis of the femoral shaft.[6,8,9] The mean angle of this lateral deviation has been reported to be 19° for cartilaginous surfaces and 16.8° for the osseous surfaces. This angle allows the tibiofemoral joint to be parallel with the ground when viewed in the coronal plane.[10,11] The sulcus angle, which reflects the depth of the trochlear groove, averages 138° ± 6° in a normal trochlea[7] and has been correlated with symptoms of patellofemoral instability.[12] Across the general population, the sulcus angle may vary considerably between individuals.[11]

Biomechanics

The trochlea functions as the counterpart to the patella in patellofemoral joint articulation. At first, as the knee transitions from full extension into flexion, the patella translates medially until the knee reaches 20° of flexion, at which point the patella engages the trochlear groove and translates an average of 11.5 mm laterally up to 90° of flexion.[13] The initial medial deflection of the patella into the trochlear groove is commonly referred to as the catching mechanism.[11] Laterally directed patellar tracking can be attributed to the normal off-axis valgus alignment of the trochlear groove relative to the femur.[13]

The patella is most susceptible to dislocation between 0° and 20° of flexion because of disengagement with the trochlea and a slack medial patellofemoral ligament restraint.[13] The dynamic traction force exerted by the quadriceps muscles is minimized in extension, which further contributes to patellar instability in this position. However, beyond 30° of flexion, the quadriceps are again able to exert a sufficient traction force to stabilize the patella within the trochlear groove.[11,14] In addition, in deep knee flexion, the patella becomes further stabilized to pathologic lateral displacement because of the posteriorly directed resultant force of the quadriceps muscles that ensures close contact with the lateral trochlear facet.[11,14]

THE ANATOMY AND BIOMECHANICS OF TROCHLEAR DYSPLASIA
Anatomy

Trochlear dysplasia is defined as any bony change or variation in the trochlear groove or medial or lateral facet. The defining characteristic of trochlear dysplasia is a shallow, flattened trochlea,[15] which is quantitatively defined as an increased sulcus angle. A sulcus angle greater than 145° is considered dysplastic and is generally defined as a shallow trochlea.[3,7,16] In addition, abnormal patellar tilt and patellar height may also contribute to an abnormally increased sulcus angle.[12] As the sulcus angle increases, the depth of the trochlear groove relative to the medial and lateral facets decreases. In one study, patients presenting with symptomatic patellar instability had a reported depth of 2.3 ± 1.8 mm compared with a depth of 7.8 ± 1.5 mm in an asymptomatic control group.[3]

Biomechanics

Abnormal bony anatomy associated with a dysplastic trochlea alters the biomechanics of the patellofemoral joint substantially because of a lack of inherent bony stability. A dysplastic trochlea is strongly correlated with a history of patellofemoral joint instability.[3,17] A shallow trochlea permits unbounded and pathologic lateral displacement of the patella.[18] The decreased resistance to lateral patellar translation resulting from a shallow lateral facet places increased stress on the medial soft tissue restraints, primarily the medial patellofemoral ligament (MPFL).[15] It has been reported that a dysplastic trochlea is more likely to result in lateral patellar displacement than either a ruptured medial retinaculum or a vastus medialis obliquus release.[18] For this reason, when patellar instability is suspected, it is important to assess trochlear morphology as the possible cause because of its significant contributions to patellar stability.

DIAGNOSIS OF TROCHLEAR DYSPLASIA
History and Physical Examination

When evaluating patients with suspected trochlear dysplasia, it is essential to begin by obtaining a detailed history to discern whether the presenting symptoms are the result of an acute dislocation or chronic instability. Inspection of the knee may reveal a patella that sits laterally and proximal relative to the trochlea. Other changes such as bruising, swelling, or effusion should also be assessed. On physical examination, the clinician must check patellar mobility to test for excessive laxity. The patella can be separated into 4 equal sections, also known as quadrants, which divide the patella into quarters from medial to lateral. When a laterally directed force is applied to the patella, normal patellar mobility should remain within 2 quadrants compared with the resting state.

The patellar apprehension test is also an excellent indicator of patellofemoral instability.[19,20] The patellar apprehension test is performed by applying a laterally directed force on the patella as the knee transitions from full extension into flexion. This test functionally mimics a lateral patellar dislocation.[21] A positive test is defined as visible apprehension or activation of the quadriceps muscles. The diagnostic accuracy of this test is high, as seen in one series with a reported sensitivity of 100%, a specificity of 88.4%, a positive predictive value of 89.2%, a negative predictive value of 100%, and an accuracy of 94.1%.[21]

Although widely used, the interobserver reliability of the physical examination for assessing patellofemoral joint instability is poor and the intraobserver reliability is only moderate.[22] Even when a thorough history is elicited and a comprehensive physical examination is performed, trochlear dysplasia is challenging to diagnose and is best evaluated using imaging, which renders a more comprehensive and objective assessment of trochlear morphology.

Radiographic Evaluation

Previous studies have described the use of lateral radiographs for the assessment of abnormal trochlear morphology.[3,23] Lateral radiographs are useful for classifying abnormal trochlear morphology according to the widely used Dejour classification system.[3,24] In the Dejour system, trochlear dysplasia is classified using lateral radiographs as types A through D depending on the presence of a crossing sign, supratrochlear spur, and/or a double contour (**Figs. 1** and **2**). The Dejour grade not only helps to characterize the various manifestations of trochlear dysplasia but may also be useful for formulating a preoperative plan uniquely tailored to each patient.

In addition to lateral radiographs, axial radiographs captured with the knee in 30° of flexion enable assessment of the sulcus angle and the depth of the trochlear groove (**Fig. 3**).[23] A sulcus angle of 145° or greater indicates a dysplastic trochlea.[3] Although the sulcus angle is widely used and well described in the literature, it has several

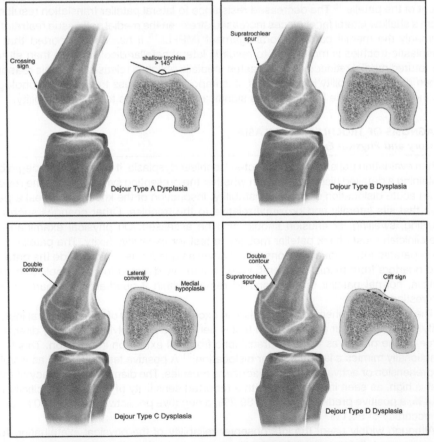

Fig. 1. Lateral radiographic views and axial cross sections representing the 4-part Dejour classification system for trochlear dysplasia. (*Courtesy of* the Steadman Philippon Research Institute, Vail, CO; with permission.)

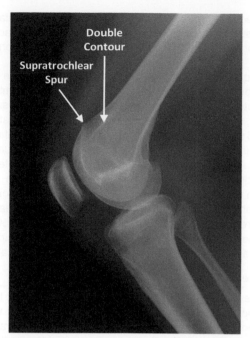

Fig. 2. Features of trochlear dysplasia shown on a lateral radiograph: the double contour and supratrochlear spur.

potential weaknesses. The sulcus angle describes the flatness of the trochlear groove in the transverse plane, but it does not describe side-to-side differences in the inclination of the medial and lateral trochlear facets.[25] For example, a shallow trochlear groove with the same sulcus angle measurement may be caused by a shallow

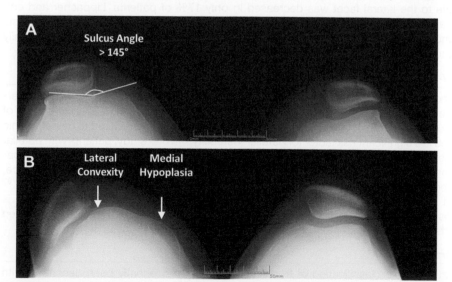

Fig. 3. Sunrise radiographic views showing the Dejour classification system for trochlear dysplasia: (A) dysplasia type A with a shallow sulcus angle (right knee); (B) dysplasia type C with lateral convexity and medial hypoplasia of the trochlea (left knee).

inclination of the medial and/or lateral facets. Therefore, the medial and lateral trochlear inclination measurements, which describe the inclination of the medial and lateral facets, have been proposed to more precisely characterize abnormal trochlear bony morphology.

Numerous other quantitative radiographic measurements have been described in the literature for trochlear dysplasia. Among the various quantitative radiographic methods for characterizing trochlear morphology, including the sulcus angle, lateral trochlear inclination, and medial trochlear inclination, a flattened lateral trochlear inclination is considered the best predictor of both lateral patellar displacement and lateral patellofemoral articular cartilage lesions.[25,26] However, these quantitative measurements do not correlate with the Dejour 4-grade classification system and may be unreliable when performed for high grades of dysplasia.[27,28] In cases of extreme trochlear disorder in which a trochleoplasty is the treatment of choice, some trochlear landmarks appear amorphic on imaging, making quantitative measurements difficult to perform. Therefore, because of the strengths and weaknesses of each radiographic diagnostic technique, trochlear dysplasia is best characterized using a combination of quantitative radiographic measurements and the Dejour classification system.

Magnetic Resonance Imaging

Magnetic resonance imaging (MRI) is also an important diagnostic tool to evaluate soft tissue injury and the health of the articular cartilage in patients with patellofemoral instability. In addition, MRI can be used to calculate the lateral trochlear inclination.[25,26] The lateral trochlear inclination is a measure of the angle created between a line adjacent to the posterior edges of the femoral condyles and a second line tangential to the subchondral bone of the lateral trochlear facet.[9] A shallow lateral trochlear inclination has been positively correlated with the presence of anterior knee pain.[29] On the axial view, Biedert and Bachmann[30] reported that the height of the central trochlear groove to the medial facet was decreased in 83% of patients with patellar instability. By comparison, the height of the central trochlear groove relative to the lateral facet was decreased in only 17% of patients. Lippacher and colleagues[31] reported the best overall agreement between type B Dejour dysplasia and measurements performed on MRI. By comparison, lateral radiographs generally underestimated trochlear dysplasia compared with axial MRI.

TT-TG Distance

The TT-TG distance is used to determine the degree of lateralization of the tibial tubercle in relation to the deepest part of the trochlear groove (**Fig. 4**). A TT-TG distance of more than 20 mm on computed tomography (CT) scans is considered to be pathologic and is a significant risk factor for patellar instability.[3] In one study, patients with patellar dislocation had an average TT-TG distance that was 4 mm larger than healthy patients.[32] There has been some debate as to whether to normalize the TT-TG distance, because the TT-TG distance has been shown to vary with increasing age and height.[33] At present, CT is considered the gold standard for measurement, but there is disagreement as to whether TT-TG distances measured on MRI can be considered interchangeable with those measured on CT.[34,35]

Arthroscopy

Arthroscopic classification of trochlear dysplasia has recently been described with excellent intraobserver and interobserver reliability.[36] Neiltz and colleagues described a 2-part classification system for trochlear dysplasia that could be distinguished on arthroscopic examination.[37] Neiltz type I trochlear dysplasia was defined as a flat

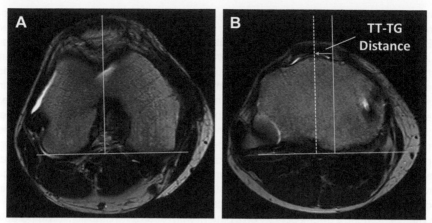

Fig. 4. (A) The measurement technique for the TT-TG distance consists of creating a posterior intercondylar line and 2 perpendicular lines to the posterior intercondylar line: one extended through the center of the deepest part of the trochlear groove and a second through the center of the patellar tendon attachment on the tibial tubercle. (B) The distance between the trochlear groove and tibial tubercle lines represents the TT-TG distance.

trochlear groove and an elevated trochlear floor. Neiltz type II trochlear dysplasia was defined as a convex proximal trochlea combined with a lateral trochlear bump. However, these types did not correspond with the standard Dejour classification system.

NATURAL HISTORY

The natural history of recurrent patellar dislocation caused by trochlear dysplasia has been well defined. For acute dislocations, Colvin and West[38] investigated nonoperative treatment after an acute lateral patellar dislocation and showed that physical therapy and bracing can be effective. However, after an acute dislocation event, the presence of trochlear dysplasia increases the risk of recurrent dislocations[39] and outcomes are worse for patients with chronic patellofemoral instability. Arnbjornsson and colleagues[40] showed poor outcomes after nonoperative treatment of chronic instability including physical therapy, with 5 of 21 knees showing degenerative changes in patients with a mean age of just 39 years. Lewallen and colleagues[41] studied the risk factors associated with development of recurrent patellar dislocation in a pediatric and adolescent population after a first-time dislocation. In these patients, recurrent instability was significantly correlated with trochlear dysplasia. Patients with open physes and trochlear dysplasia had a recurrence rate of 69%. Nonoperative management in these patients was successful in only 31% of cases. In another series, trochlear dysplasia was present in 85% of patients with recurrent instability.[3] Because patellofemoral instability is often recurrent in patients with trochlear dysplasia, surgical correction must be strongly considered when nonoperative treatment fails.

TREATMENT OPTIONS

Patellar instability in the setting of trochlear dysplasia can be problematic to treat. Patients with a history of more than one dislocation and failed conservative treatment, such as physical therapy and bracing, should consider surgical intervention. Trochleoplasty is recommended for patients with recurrent instability and trochlear dysplasia. Several techniques for trochleoplasty have been described in the literature, but the elevation of the lateral trochlear facet and the trochlear-deepening procedure are currently the most widely used.

Elevation of the lateral facet for treatment of trochlear dysplasia was first described by Albee.[42] In this procedure, an opening wedge osteotomy of the lateral facet is performed by elevating the facet with a bone wedge to effectively deepen the trochlea. There are some concerns that when the lateral facet is elevated by more than 6 mm it may increase contact pressures in the patellofemoral joint.[43] The trochlear-deepening procedure was first described by Masse[44] in 1978 before being modified by Dejour and Saggin[6] in 1987. Bereiter and Gaultier[45] also described similar procedure. In general, to perform the trochlear-deepening procedure the articular cartilage is peeled off and the subchondral bone is resected in order to recreate a normal-shaped trochlea. The deepening procedure is favored rather than the lateral facet elevation procedure because of the risk of overconstraining the patellofemoral joint and increasing the stress on the articular cartilage.

When performing a trochleoplasty on a patient with recurrent instability, it is imperative to assess the entire patellofemoral joint and to treat associated disorders concurrently. First, the medial soft tissue structures should be evaluated on MRI during the preoperative planning phase and assessed again using direct visualization during the surgery. Because the MPFL has been shown to provide up to 60% of resistance to lateral displacement of the patella,[46] anyone with recurrent instability should be considered for an MPFL reconstruction with the goal of restoring normal patellofemoral kinematics.

Patients with patella alta or a TT-TG distance greater than 20 mm may require a tibial tubercle osteotomy. A distalization of the tubercle is recommended for patients presenting with patella alta. A medialization and/or an anteriorization of the tubercle is recommended for patients with a TT-TG measurement greater than 20 mm to decrease contact pressures on the lateral trochlear and patellar facets. In light of a recent study that reported a decreased TT-TG in young and short patients,[33] some patients with a TT-TG distance only slightly less than the traditional 20 mm threshold may still be considered candidates for a tibial tubercle osteotomy at the discretion of the treating surgeon.

INDICATIONS FOR A TROCHLEOPLASTY

First-time acute patellar dislocations should be treated nonoperatively in a brace. Patients with a history of chronic dislocations with Dejour type A trochlear dysplasia should undergo a medial-sided soft tissue reconstruction rather than a trochleoplasty. A sulcus-deepening trochleoplasty is recommended for Dejour types B, C, and D dysplasia. Specifically, type C can also be considered for a lateral facet–elevating trochleoplasty, although this remains controversial because of the theoretic risk of increasing contact pressures in the patellofemoral joint. An MPFL reconstruction should be performed in conjunction with any trochleoplasty procedure.[6]

A trochleoplasty is contraindicated in patients with open physes. Instead, a medial soft tissue procedure such as an MPFL reconstruction should be proposed as a safe surgical alternative in these patients. In addition, a trochleoplasty is also contraindicated in patients with diffuse patellofemoral arthritis because of a significant risk of increasing pain levels.

SULCUS-DEEPENING TROCHLEOPLASTY AND MPFL RECONSTRUCTION
Surgical Procedure

The patient is induced under general anesthesia and positioned supine on the operating table. A high thigh tourniquet is placed and a thorough examination under anesthesia is performed to confirm the preoperative diagnosis. An anterior midline incision is created along with a medial parapatellar arthrotomy.

The course of the MPFL is followed along the distal edge of the vastus medialis obliquus (VMO) with a sharp dissection medially, and the adductor magnus tendon is identified. Using the adductor magnus tendon as a landmark, the adductor tubercle and medial epicondyle are identified. The femoral attachment of the MPFL is located at a point 1.9 mm anterior and 3.8 mm distal to the adductor tubercle[47] and 2 suture anchors are placed in this location. The MPFL attachment on the patella is then identified, which is approximately 41% from the proximal pole, and a guide pin is placed transversely across the patella. A cannulated 5-mm reamer is used to ream a tunnel across the patella, and a passing suture is placed through the tunnel. As an alternative, for a small patella, a small trough can be created with a bur and a cortical button device can be used to secure the graft to the medial patella.

If an autograft is used, the semitendinosus tendon is identified within the pes anserine bursa and harvested with an open tendon stripper. The graft is then tubularized and prepared on the back table. The graft should be at least 16 cm in length.

Attention is then turned to exposing the trochlea (**Fig. 5**). A scalpel is used to elevate the periosteum 5 to 6 mm away from the articular cartilage margins along the proximal femur. From medial to lateral, 3 Kirschner wires (K-wires) are placed parallel to the joint, 3 to 4 mm posterior to the subchondral bone of the trochlea with the use of an anterior cruciate ligament guide (**Fig. 6**). An osteotome is then used to connect the K-wires in a proximal to distal fashion down to the sulcus terminalis. Once the articular cartilage is elevated from the femur, the osteotome is used to carefully create a V shape in the subchondral bone. Once this is completed, a high-speed burr is used to undermine the subchondral bone on the articular cartilage flap to help press the cartilage margins into position (**Fig. 7**). The flap is then pushed into the newly created trough. When good trochlear position is confirmed, the flap is secured with 2 biocompression screws into both the medial and lateral trochlear facets.

Next, the MPFL graft is passed transversely across the previously created channel along the normal course of the native MPFL deep to the superficial layer of the medial retinaculum, just distal to the VMO, and is tied to the suture anchors at the femoral attachment. Using the passing suture in the patella, the graft is pulled through the patella and brought back and tied on itself in a neutral position in the trochlea at 40° of knee flexion while being careful not to overmedialize the patella. Once the graft has a few sutures in place, the patella is tested with lateral translation at varying degrees of

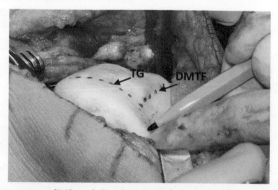

Fig. 5. The trochlear groove (TG) and distal aspect of the medial trochlear facet (DMTF) outlined before performing a trochleoplasty procedure (left knee).

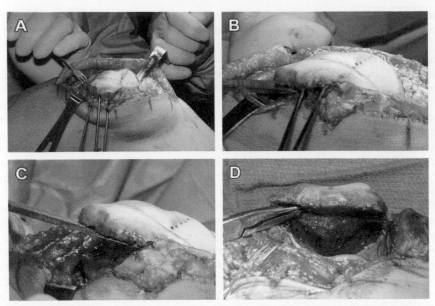

Fig. 6. (*A*) A trochleoplasty is performed by making a parapatellar longitudinal incision and placing guide pins underneath and parallel to the trochlear groove; (*B*) an osteotome is used to free the trochlea by following the guide pins; (*C*) the trochlea is elevated; (*D*) bone is resected below the trochlea to create a deepened sulcus (left knee).

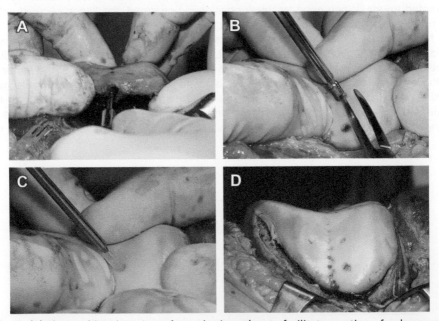

Fig. 7. (*A*) The trochleoplasty is performed using a bur to facilitate creation of a decreased sulcus angle; a tap (*B*) is used to prepare attachment sites for bioabsorbable screws (*C*), which secure the deepened trochlea as it heals; (*D*) the completed sulcus-deepening trochleoplasty (left knee).

Table 1
Review of outcomes after trochleoplasty

Author Ref, Year	Number of Knees	Mean and Range of Follow-Up (mo)	Outcomes
Goutallier et al,[51] 2002	12	48 (24–72)	67% satisfaction rate
Schöttle et al,[53] 2005	19	36 (24–48)	16 of 19 knees improved subjectively Kujala score increased from 56 to 80 points
Verdonk et al,[49] 2005	13	18 (8–34)	Larsen-Lauridsen scoring system: 7 patients scored poor, 3 fair, 3 good; 77% of patients reported good or very good results subjectively
Donell et al,[54] 2006	17	36 (12–108)	Seven patients were very satisfied, 6 were satisfied, and 2 were disappointed. Kujala score average of 48 (range 13–75) to 75 (range 51–98) out of 100
von Knoch et al,[50] 2006	48	100 (48–168)	Mean Kujala score, 94.9 (range, 80–100)
Fucentese et al,[55] 2007	17	36 (24–48)	Trochleoplasty created more normal anatomy
Utting et al,[4] 2008	59	24 (12–58)	92.6% of patients satisfied Oxford knee score, 26 (12–43) to 19 (12–44) WOMAC score, 23 (12–35) to 17 (12–34) IKDC score, 54 (26–89) to 72 (23–100) Kujala score, 62 (29–92) to 76 (26–100) Lysholm score, 57 (25–91) to 78 (30–100)
Zaki et al,[56] 2010	27	54 (12–72)	33% had residual symptoms Lysholm score improved from a mean preoperative score of 54 (range, 32–61) to a mean 83 (good to excellent) in 19 (70%) and 65–83 (fair) in 8 (30%) knees
Thaunat et al,[57] 2011	19	34 (12–71)	Kujala score, 80 ($\pm$17) KOOS score, 70 ($\pm$18) IKDC score, 67 ($\pm$17)
Faruqui et al,[20] 2012	6	68.3	WOMAC score increased by 20% KOOS score increased by 74.50%
Koch et al,[58] 2011	2	24	Stable patella with correct tracking Both patients rated their result as excellent
Dejour et al,[59] 2013	24	66 (24–191)	No patellar redislocation Kujala score improved from 44 (25–73) to 81 (53–100)
Nelitz et al,[36] 2013	26	30 (24–42)	Kujala scores improved from 79 to 96 IKDC scores improved from 74 to 90 VAS scores improved from 3 to 1 95.7% of patients were satisfied or very satisfied No recurrent dislocation occurred after surgery
Ntagiopoulos et al,[60] 2013	31	84 (24–108)	IKDC score improved from 51 (range, 25–80) to 82 (range, 40–100) Kujala score improved from 59 (range, 28–81) to 87 (range, 49–100)

Kujala score refers to the Kujala scale for patellofemoral pain.

Abbreviations: IKDC, International Knee Documentation Committee; KOOS, Knee Injury and Osteoarthritis Outcome Score; VAS, Visual Analog Pain Scale; WOMAC, Western Ontario and McMaster Universities Osteoarthritis Index.

knee flexion to confirm restoration of an adequate restraint to lateral translation with no evidence of overtightening medially. Once this is confirmed, the remaining sutures are secured. In addition, the arthrotomy is copiously irrigated and closed. Steri-Strips and a sterile dressing are placed over the incision, and the knee is placed in an immobilizer.

Postoperative Rehabilitation

Patients should remain non–weight bearing for 6 weeks. A continuous passive motion (CPM) machine is used to cycle the knee from 0° to 30° of flexion in order to minimize the risk of arthrofibrosis and to maintain articular cartilage viability. The CPM should be used for 6 to 8 hours per day for a total of 6 weeks after surgery. Passive range of motion should be limited from 0° to 90° of flexion for the first 2 weeks and increased as tolerated thereafter. Return to normal levels of activity generally occurs after 6 to 9 months.

Complications

Postsurgical complications include deep vein thrombosis, infection, and residual skin numbness. Complications specific to trochleoplasty include trochlear cartilage damage, patellar incongruence, and overcorrection.[6] Articular cartilage cell viability is also a concern following trochleoplasty. In one study, Schöttle and colleagues[48] investigated histologic changes in the trochlear articular cartilage following a trochleoplasty procedure in 13 patients. Using confocal microscopy and histologic examination, the articular cartilage appeared normal after undergoing a trochleoplasty procedure. However, small changes were noted in the calcified layer, which requires further investigation. Overall, the results of this study suggest there is minimal risk of cartilage damage after trochleoplasty.

Some patients also experience arthrofibrosis after surgery, although reports on the incidence of this complication are mixed and likely vary as a function of range of motion exercises during postoperative rehabilitation. Verdonk and colleagues[49] reported 5 of 13 patients experienced arthrofibrosis after trochleoplasty, whereas von Knoch and colleagues[50] reported that all of the patients in their cohort had gained full range of motion by the final follow-up with no signs of arthrofibrosis. Early range of motion is critical and may decrease the risk of patients developing postoperative arthrofibrosis.

OUTCOMES AFTER TROCHLEOPLASTY

Outcomes after trochleoplasty with or without MPFL reconstruction are mixed. Previous studies have reported a patient satisfaction rate as low as 67%[51] to as high as 95.7%.[36] Although many outcome measures have been used in the literature to describe results after trochleoplasty, only the Fulkerson and Lysholm scales have been reported to be reliable and valid for differentiating between patients with and without recurrent patellar instability.[52] A summary of outcomes after sulcus-deepening trochleoplasty with or without MPFL reconstruction is presented in **Table 1**.

SUMMARY

The diagnosis and treatment of chronic patellar instability caused by trochlear dysplasia can be challenging. A dysplastic trochlea leads to biomechanical and kinematic changes that often require surgical correction when symptomatic. In the past, trochlear dysplasia was classified using the 4-part Dejour classification system. More recently, new classification systems have been proposed. Future studies are needed to investigate long-term outcomes after trochleoplasty.

REFERENCES

1. Fithian DC, Paxton EW, Stone ML, et al. Epidemiology and natural history of acute patellar dislocation. Am J Sports Med 2004;32:1114–21.
2. Mehta VM, Inoue M, Nomura E, et al. An algorithm guiding the evaluation and treatment of acute primary patellar dislocations. Sports Med Arthrosc 2007;15(2):78–81.
3. Dejour H, Walch G, Nove-Josserand L, et al. Factors of patellar instability: an anatomic radiographic study. Knee Surg Sports Traumatol Arthrosc 1994;2:19–26.
4. Utting MR, Mulford JS, Eldridge JD. A prospective evaluation of trochleoplasty for the treatment of patellofemoral dislocation and instability. J Bone Joint Surg Br 2008;90:180–5.
5. O'Brien M. Clinical anatomy of the patellofemoral joint. Int J Sports Med 2001;2:1–8.
6. Dejour D, Saggin P. The sulcus deepening trochleoplasty – the Lyon's procedure. Int Orthop 2010;34:311–6.
7. Tecklenburg K, Dejour D, Hoser C, et al. Bony and cartilaginous anatomy of the patellofemoral joint. Knee Surg Sports Traumatol Arthrosc 2006;14:235–40.
8. Eckhoff DG, Burke BJ, Dwyer TF, et al. Sulcus morphology of the distal femur. Clin Orthop 1996;331:23–8.
9. Shih YF, Bull AM, Amis AA. The cartilaginous and osseous geometry of the femoral trochlear groove. Knee Surg Sports Traumatol Arthrosc 2004;12:300–6.
10. Shih YF, Bull AM, Amis AA. Geometry of the distal femur: comparison of the cartilaginous and osseous characteristics of the trochlear groove. Knee Surg Sports Traumatol Arthrosc 2003;12:300–6.
11. Amis AA. Current concepts on anatomy and biomechanics of patellar stability. Sports Med Arthrosc 2007;15:48–56.
12. Davies AP, Costa ML, Shepstone L, et al. The sulcus angle and malalignment of the extensor mechanism of the knee. J Bone Joint Surg Br 2000;82(8):1162–6.
13. Amis AA, Senavongse W, Bull AM. Patellofemoral kinematics during knee flexion-extension: an in vitro study. J Orthop Res 2006;24:2201–11.
14. Amis AA, Farahmand F. Biomechanics masterclass: extensor mechanism of the knee. Curr Orthop 1996;10:102–9.
15. Bollier M, Fulkerson JP. The role of trochlear dysplasia in patellofemoral instability. J Am Acad Orthop Surg 2011;19:8–16.
16. van Huyssteen AL, Hendrix MR, Barnett AJ, et al. Cartilage-bone mismatch in the dysplastic trochlea: an MRI study. J Bone Joint Surg Br 2006;88:688–91.
17. Eckhoff DG, Montgomery WK, Stamm ER, et al. Location of the femoral sulcus in the osteoarthritic knee. J Arthroplasty 1996;11(2):163–5.
18. Senavongse W, Amis AA. The effects of articular, retinacular, or muscular deficiencies on patellofemoral joint stability. J Bone Joint Surg Br 2005;87:577–82.
19. Sallay PI, Poggi J, Speer KP, et al. Acute dislocation of the patella. A correlative pathoanatomic study. Am J Sports Med 1996;24:52–60.
20. Faruqui S, Bollier M, Wolf B, et al. Outcomes after trochleoplasty. Iowa Orthop J 2012;32:196–206.
21. Ahmad CS, McCarthy M, Gomez JA, et al. The moving patellar apprehension test for lateral patellar instability. Am J Sports Med 2009;37:791–6.
22. Smith TO, Clark A, Neda S, et al. The intra- and inter-observer reliability of the physical examination methods used to assess patients with patellofemoral joint instability. Knee 2012;19:404–10.
23. Malghem J, Maldague B. Depth insufficiency of the proximal trochlear groove on lateral radiographs of the knee: relation to patellar dislocation. Radiology 1989;170:507–10.

24. Dejour D, Le Coultre B. Osteotomies in patellofemoral instabilities. Sports Med Arthrosc 2007;15:40.
25. Stefanik JJ, Roemer FW, Zumwalt AC, et al. Association between measures of trochlear morphology and structural features of patellofemoral joint osteoarthritis on MRI: the MOST study. J Orthop Res 2012;30:1–8.
26. Stefanik JJ, Zumwalt AC, Segal NA, et al. Association between measures of patella height, morphologic features of the trochlea, and patellofemoral joint alignment: the MOST study. Clin Orthop Relat Res 2013;471:2641–8.
27. Nelitz M, Lippacher S, Reichel H, et al. Evaluation of trochlear dysplasia using MRI: correlation between the classification system of Dejour and objective parameters of trochlear dysplasia. Knee Surg Sports Traumatol Arthrosc 2014;22(1):120–7.
28. Carrillon Y, Abidi H, Dejour D, et al. Patellar instability: assessment on MR images by measuring the lateral trochlear inclination-initial experience. Radiology 2000;216:582–5.
29. Keser S, Savranlar A, Bayar A, et al. Is there a relationship between anterior knee pain and femoral trochlear dysplasia? Assessment of lateral trochlear inclination by magnetic resonance imaging. Knee Surg Sports Traumatol Arthrosc 2008;16:911–5.
30. Biedert RM, Bachmann M. Anterior-posterior trochlear measurements of normal and dysplastic trochlea by axial magnetic resonance imaging. Knee Surg Sports Traumatol Arthrosc 2009;17:1225–30.
31. Lippacher S, Dejour D, Elsharkawi M, et al. Observer agreement on the Dejour trochlear dysplasia classification: a comparison of true lateral radiographs and axial magnetic resonance images. Am J Sports Med 2012;40:837–43.
32. Balcarek P, Ammon J, Frosch S, et al. Magnetic resonance imaging characteristics of the medial patellofemoral ligament lesion in acute lateral patellar dislocations considering trochlear dysplasia, patella alta, and tibial tuberosity-trochlear groove distance. Arthroscopy 2010;26:926–35.
33. Pennock AT, Alam M, Bastrom T. Variation in tibial tubercle-trochlear groove measurement as a function of age, sex, size, and patellar instability. Am J Sports Med 2014;42(2):389–93.
34. Schoettle PB, Zanetti M, Seifert B, et al. The tibial tuberosity-trochlear groove distance; a comparative study between CT and MRI scanning. Knee 2006;13:26–31.
35. Camp CL, Stuart MJ, Krych AJ, et al. CT and MRI measurements of tibial tubercle-trochlear groove distances are not equivalent in patients with patellar instability. Am J Sports Med 2013;41:1835–40.
36. Nelitz M, Dreyhaupt J, Lippacher S. Combined trochleoplasty and medial patellofemoral ligament reconstruction for recurrent patellar dislocations in severe trochlear dysplasia: a minimum 2-year follow-up study. Am J Sports Med 2013;41:1005–12.
37. Nelitz M, Lippacher S. Arthroscopic evaluation of trochlear dysplasia as an aid in decision making for the treatment of patellofemoral instability. Knee Surg Sports Traumatol Arthrosc 2013. [Epub ahead of print].
38. Colvin AC, West RV. Patellar instability. J Bone Joint Surg Am 2008;90:2751–62.
39. Cash J, Hughston JC. Treatment of acute patellar dislocation. Am J Sports Med 1988;16:244–9.
40. Arnbjornsson A, Egund N, Ryding O, et al. The natural history of recurrent dislocation of the patella: long-term results of conservative and operative treatment. J Bone Joint Surg Br 1992;72:140–2.
41. Lewallen LW, McIntosh AL, Dahm DL. Predictors of recurrent instability after acute patellofemoral dislocation in pediatric and adolescent patients. Am J Sports Med 2013;41:575–81.

42. Albee FH. The bone graft wedge in the treatment of habitual dislocation of the patella. Med Rec 1915;88:257–9.
43. Kuroda R, Kambic H, Valdevit A, et al. Distribution of patellofemoral joint pressures after femoral trochlear osteotomy. Knee Surg Sports Traumatol Arthrosc 2002;10:33–7.
44. Masse Y. Trochleoplasty. Restoration of the intercondylar groove in subluxations and dislocations of the patella. Rev Chir Orthop Reparatrice Appar Mot 1978;64: 3–17.
45. Bereiter HG, Gautier E. Die Trochleoplastik ale chirurgishe Therapie der rezidivierenden Patellauxation bei Trochleodysplasie des Femurs. Arthroskopie 1994; 7:281–6.
46. Desio SM, Burks RT, Bachus KN. Soft tissue restraints to lateral patellar translation in the human knee. Am J Sports Med 1998;26(1):59–65.
47. LaPrade RF, Engebretsen AH, Ly TV, et al. The anatomy of the medial part of the knee. J Bone Joint Surg Am 2007;89(9):2000–10.
48. Schottle PB, Schell H, Duda G, et al. Cartilage viability after trochleoplasty. Knee Surg Sports Traumatol Arthrosc 2007;15:161–7.
49. Verdonk R, Jansegers E, Stuyts B. Trochleoplasty in dysplastic knee trochlea. Knee Surg Sports Traumatol Arthrosc 2005;13:529–33.
50. von Knoch F, Böhm T, Bürgi ML, et al. Trochleoplasty for recurrent patellar dislocation in association with trochlear dysplasia. A 4- to 14-year follow-up study. J Bone Joint Surg Br 2006;88:1331–5.
51. Paxton EW, Fithian DC, Stone ML, et al. The reliability and validity of knee-specific and general health instruments in assessing acute patellar dislocation outcomes. Am J Sports Med 2003;31:487–92.
52. Goutallier D, Raou D, Van Driessche S. Retro-trochlear wedge reduction trochleoplasty for the treatment of painful patella syndrome with protruding trochleae. Technical note and early results. Rev Chir Orthop Reparatrice Appar Mot 2002; 88(7):678–85.
53. Schöttle PB, Fucentese SF, Pfirrmann C, et al. Trochleoplasty for patellar instability due to trochlear dysplasia: a minimum 2-year clinical and radiological follow-up of 19 knees. Acta Orthop 2005;76:693–8.
54. Donell ST, Joseph G, Hing CB, et al. Modified Dejour trochleoplasty for severe dysplasia: operative technique and early clinical results. Knee 2006;13:266–73.
55. Fucentese SF, Schöttle PB, Pfirrmann CW, et al. CT changes after trochleoplasty for symptomatic trochlear dysplasia. Knee Surg Sports Traumatol Arthrosc 2007;15:168–74.
56. Zaki SH, Rae PJ. Femoral trochleoplasty for recurrent patellar instability: a modified surgical technique and its medium-term results. Curr Orthop Pract 2010;21: 153–7.
57. Thaunat M, Bessiere C, Pujol N, et al. Recession wedge trochleoplasty as an additional procedure in the surgical treatment of patellar instability with major trochlear dysplasia: early results. Orthop Traumatol Surg Res 2011;97:833–45.
58. Koch PP, Fuchs B, Meyer DC, et al. Closing wedge patellar osteotomy in combination with trochleoplasty. Acta Orthop Belg 2011;77:116–21.
59. Dejour D, Byn P, Ntagiopoulos PG. The Lyon's sulcus-deepening trochleoplasty in previous unsuccessful patellofemoral surgery. Int Orthop 2013;37:433–9.
60. Ntagiopoulos PG, Byn P, Dejour D. Midterm results of comprehensive surgical reconstruction including sulcus-deepening trochleoplasty in recurrent patellar dislocations with high-grade trochlear dysplasia. Am J Sports Med 2013;41: 998–1004.

Patellofemoral Arthroplasty in the Athlete

Jack Farr, MD[a],*, Elizabeth Arendt, MD[b], Diane Dahm, MD[c], Jake Daynes, DO[d]

KEYWORDS

- Patellofemoral • Arthroplasty • Athlete • Sports participation recommendations

KEY POINTS

- Despite an increasing number of patient athletes undergoing patellofemoral arthroplasty (PFA) for isolated/end-stage arthritis, no postoperative sports participation recommendations exist.
- Patients undergoing PFA can be divided into the 3 groups with overlapping disease characteristics: those with patellofemoral dysplasia, traumatic arthritis, and a predisposition for arthritis in the patellofemoral joint.
- Current PFA techniques and implants are related to decreased implant failure and improved clinical outcomes.
- High impact sports may lead to an increase in catastrophic failure and polyethylene wear.
- The benefits of maintaining an active lifestyle are well documented and can be realized even after PFA.
- Lower-impact sports, such as golf, swimming, doubles tennis, and skiing, are acceptable activities after PFA.

INTRODUCTION

Workplace, societal, and governmental policy changes since the mid-20th century have led to more free time, more athletic options beginning at early ages, more female participation in sports, and increasing obesity. Patellofemoral arthritis is multifactorial and is more prevalent in women and in those with high patellofemoral loading (eg, from athletics and obesity).[1,2] As a result, more patients are presenting with end-stage patellofemoral arthritis at earlier ages, which is increasingly being treated with patellofemoral arthroplasty (PFA).[3] However, these patients often desire to continue with some level

Authors have no commercial or financial disclosures.
[a] Department of Orthopaedic Surgery, Cartilage Restoration Center of Indiana, 1260 Innovation Parkway, Suite 100, Greenwood, IN 46143, USA; [b] Department of Orthopaedic Surgery, University of Minnesota, 2450 Riverside Avenue, Suite R200, Minneapolis, MN 55454, USA; [c] Department of Orthopaedic Surgery, Mayo Clinic, 200 First Street Southwest, Rochester, MN 55905, USA; [d] Department of Orthopaedic Surgery, OrthoIndy, 1260 Innovation Parkway, Suite 100, Greenwood, IN 46143, USA
* Corresponding author.
E-mail address: indyknee@hotmail.com

of sporting activities. The goal of the surgeon is to allow the highest postoperative activity level, with safety being paramount. Unfortunately, current guidelines for sports participation after arthroplasty are based primarily on literature for total joint arthroplasty, which is largely derived from laboratory findings and level 5 evidence.[4]

THE PATIENT

Selecting the appropriate patient for PFA begins with documenting whether the patellofemoral arthritis is both isolated and end-stage. Patellofemoral arthritis is not uncommon. Prevalence data suggest that 10% to 20% of patients who are candidates for arthroplasty have isolated patellofemoral degenerative joint disease.[5] This group comprises 3 patient types with overlapping disease characteristics: those with (1) patellofemoral dysplasia, often associated with a remote history of instability; (2) posttraumatic arthritis; and (3) normal anatomy with a probable genetic predisposition for degenerative joint disease first presenting at the patellofemoral compartment.[6] Those with recurrent instability often stop participating in sports for fear of patella instability events, whereas those with posttraumatic arthritis and/or a genetic predisposition for arthritis have gradually decreased their sporting activities as their arthritic symptoms have increased.

Once the patellofemoral pain is resolved postoperatively, many patients want to resume their preoperative sporting activity. Some may even want to start new, higher-level activities now that pain is not a limitation.[7] Based on the published activity recommendations for partial and total knee arthroplasty, beginning a new skilled sport (involving unfamiliar technique, direction change and complex form) after arthroplasty is not advisable.[4]

THE IMPLANT

Patellofemoral arthroplasty has been available almost as long as total knee arthroplasty (TKA). Just as with TKA, initial problems occurred, not only with component design but also with component materials. First-generation PFAs had problems with both wear and patellar stability, but surprisingly, not with mechanical loosening.[8] Second- and now third-generation PFA implants have addressed these initial issues and are associated with improved clinical outcomes.[9,10] Most current patellar implants are all-polyethylene components with multiple pegs that are either dome- or oval dome-shaped. The polyethylene is highly durable and not metal-backed, which leads to very low wear and loosening rates. The trochlear components match the radius of curvature of the patellar component in the axial plane and are typically based on anthropomorphic "normal" trochleas for the sagittal profile. With multiple peg fixation typical also on the femoral component, these components also have excellent fixation and low loosening rates.[10–13] These changes in design have undoubtedly improved patient outcomes. It has even been suggested that the most common mode of failure of PFA is tibiofemoral arthritis.[14]

THE PATELLOFEMORAL PREPARATION

Minimally invasive surgery (MIS) had brief popularity in knee arthroplasty surgery. For PFA, the goal never focused on MIS per se, but rather bone-sparing surgery. All third-generation PFAs have trochlear components that remove minimal bone from the femur and allow (easy) conversion to a primary TKA.[15] The patellar bone preparation is similar to that for TKA. Because the patients are often younger (especially in the subset desiring increased sport activities), the goal is to preserve as much bone stock as possible to allow future revisions and avoid (potential) patellar fractures.[16] The literature suggests that patellar bone stock of less than 12 mm thickness places the patient at increased risk of patellar fracture.[17] Therefore, care must be taken to avoid overresection of bone. However, the work of Bengs and Scott[18] showed that the concerns about patellar "overstuffing" are largely unfounded, because their study showed that even with an exaggerated composite thickness of the patellofemoral components, minimal loss of flexion occurred. With the 2 goals of allowing revision to a primary component and avoiding fracture in the young athlete, leaving a substantial thickness of patella makes intuitive sense, although this has not been proven.

WHY AVOID CERTAIN SPORTS
Catastrophic Failure

Sports may be categorized with respect to the level of loading. The TKA literature has grouped sports according to perceived loading, and suggests that they can be categorized as acceptable-, moderate-, and high-risk.[4,19] In the category of catastrophic injury, the risks to PFA are predominantly fracture and dislocation. Fractures can never be totally avoided, but the 2 major risks may be mitigated by maintaining adequate patellar bone stock and avoiding the typical mechanisms of patellar fracture: high extensor loads (eg, eccentric landing from a jump) and direct impact (eg, fall).[17] Although sports by nature are never fully predictable, the common mechanisms of injury for each sport are well-known; that is, basketball has high eccentric loading, soccer has high direction-change forces, volleyball at certain positions can have repetitive direct impacts, and golf, running, and cycling have a low probability of these mechanisms.[20]

Polyethylene Wear

Although component wear by definition would include the metal trochlear component, with the current all-polyethylene patellar buttons, trochlear component wear is not a clinical factor in the human lifespan. Patellar polyethylene wear is dictated by similar factors as for standard TKA. That is, wear is linearly related to cycles (steps) and nonlinearly related to stress (force per unit area of contact).[21] Although polyethylene wear now occurs to a much lesser degree with improved material/material treatment, it still occurs.[22] With the typical patellar button thickness, thinning of the component would rarely be the reason for failure. Rather, it is the wear debris that may lead to failure. The microscopic and submicroscopic particles may cause a white cell reaction that releases cytokines, which are destructive at the bone-cement interface, leading to loosening.[21,23] Despite this theoretical concern, osteolysis and subsequent component loosening seem to be more of a concern in TKA than PFA.[22,24] Loading that leads to primary loosening at the implant-cement or cement-bone interface has not been reported in second-generation PFA components, although only mid-term results are currently available.[22,25,26]

Progression of arthritis in the tibiofemoral compartments seems to be independent of the PFA, and most dependent on genetics, tibiofemoral alignment, weight, activity, and loading.[22,24] If minimal tibiofemoral chondrosis is present, then the other factors may be discussed with the patient preoperatively. If the surgeon and patient agree that tibiofemoral degeneration is inevitable in the intermediate/distant future, both may agree that PFA is a bridging surgery to TKA.[7,16] That is, patients can enjoy the superior kinematics of PFA over TKA for years while postponing their primary TKA.

WHY ALLOW SPORTS

Time on earth is limited, and how to optimize one's time is a personal decision. As is often quoted, "pain is inevitable, suffering is optional." The pain of patellofemoral

Table 1
Results of the Knee Society Surveys

Allowed	1999	2005	Allowed with Experience	1999	2005	No Consensus	1999	2005	Not Recommended	1999	2005
Bowling	✓	✓	Canoeing	✓		Square dancing	✓		Baseball	✓	
Stationary cycling	✓	✓	Road cycling	✓		Fencing	✓	✓	Basketball	✓	✓
Ballroom dancing	✓	✓	Hiking	✓		Roller skating	✓	✓	Football	✓	✓
Golf	✓	✓	Rowing	✓	✓	Downhill skiing	✓		Gymnastics	✓	
Horseback riding	✓		Ice skating	✓	✓	Weight lifting	✓		Handball	✓	
Shuffleboard	✓	✓	Cross-country skiing	✓	✓	Baseball		✓	Hockey	✓	✓
Swimming	✓	✓	Stationary skiing	✓	✓	Gymnastics		✓	Jogging	✓	
Normal walking	✓	✓	Doubles tennis	✓	✓	Handball		✓	Rock climbing	✓	
Canoeing		✓	Speed walking	✓		Hockey		✓	Soccer	✓	✓
Road cycling		✓	Weight machine	✓		Rock climbing		✓	Squash/Racquetball	✓	
Square dancing		✓	Horseback riding		✓	Squash/Racquetball		✓	Singles tennis	✓	
Hiking		✓	Downhill skiing		✓	Singles tennis		✓	Volleyball	✓	✓
Speed walking		✓				Weight machine		✓			

This table is constructed to accurately compare the 1999 and 2005 Knee Society Surveys. The 1999 survey asked about croquet (allowed), horseshoes (allowed), shooting (allowed), and lacrosse (not recommended), which were not included in the 2005 survey. The 1999 survey asked about high-impact aerobics (not recommended) and low-impact aerobics (allowed with experience). The 2005 survey combined these activities and asked about aerobics (allowed with experience). The 2005 survey asked about yoga (allowed with experience), which was not included in the 1999 survey.

From Healy WL, Sharma S, Schwartz B, et al. Athletic activity after total joint arthroplasty. J Bone Joint Surg Am 2008;90:2250, with permission; and *Data from* Healy WL, Iorio R, Lemos MJ. Athletic activity after joint replacement. Am J Sports Med 2001;29:377–88.

Table 2 Activity risk level recommendations			
Level 1: Low Risk	**Level 2: Intermediate Risk**	**Level 3: High Risk**	**Level 4: Unacceptable High Risk**
Walking	Doubles tennis	Volleyball	Football
Cycling	Skiing	Basketball	Mixed martial arts
Swimming	Running	Soccer	Rock climbing
Golf			Parkour

arthritis can be ameliorated by avoiding patellofemoral loading. To the extreme, patients could remain wheelchair-bound. However, the physical, mental, social, and economic benefits of sports and maintaining an active lifestyle have all been well documented. With this in mind, the surgeon and patient must negotiate a "contract" specifying allowed activities that avoid a high probability of catastrophic failure and minimize wear-related failure.

SUMMARY: SPORTING RECOMMENDATIONS

The highest level of evidence-based medicine for sports after TKA is level 5 (based on expert consensus opinion and the 1999 and 2005 Knee Society Surveys; **Table 1**).[4] When extrapolating the TKA recommendations (see **Table 1**) to PFA, the level of evidence is somewhat less than 5, because obtaining consensus is difficult. Therefore, the recommendations provided in **Table 2** are simply the humble suggestions of the authors.

REFERENCES

1. McAlindon TE, Snow S, Cooper C, et al. Radiographic patterns of osteoarthritis of the knee joint in the community: the importance of the patellofemoral joint. Ann Rheum Dis 1992;51:844–9.
2. Seisler AR, Sheehan FT. Normative three-dimensional patellofemoral and tibiofemoral kinematics: a dynamic, in vivo study. IEEE Trans Biomed Eng 2007;54:1333–41.
3. Walker T, Perkinson B, Mihalko WM. Patellofemoral arthroplasty: the other unicompartmental knee replacement. J Bone Joint Surg Am 2012;94:1712–20.
4. Healy WL, Sharma S, Schwartz B, et al. Athletic activity after total joint arthroplasty. J Bone Joint Surg Am 2008;90:2245–52.
5. Davies AP, Vince AS, Shepstone L, et al. The radiologic prevalence of patellofemoral osteoarthritis. Clin Orthop Relat Res 2002;(402):206–12.
6. Grelsamer RP, Dejour D, Gould J. The pathophysiology of patellofemoral arthritis. Orthop Clin North Am 2008;39:269–74, V.
7. Dahm DL, Al-Rayashi W, Dajani K, et al. Patellofemoral arthroplasty versus total knee arthroplasty in patients with isolated patellofemoral osteoarthritis. Am J Orthop 2010;39:487–91.
8. Krajca-Radcliffe JB, Coker TP. Patellofemoral arthroplasty. A 2- to 18-year followup study. Clin Orthop Relat Res 1996;(330):143–51.
9. Mihalko WM, Boachie-Adjei Y, Spang JT, et al. Controversies and techniques in the surgical management of patellofemoral arthritis. Instr Course Lect 2008;57:365–80.
10. Lonner JH. Patellofemoral arthroplasty: pros, cons, and design considerations. Clin Orthop Relat Res 2004;(428):158–65.

11. Lonner JH. Patellofemoral arthroplasty: the impact of design on outcomes. Orthop Clin North Am 2008;39:347–54, vi.
12. Farr J, Barrett D. Optimizing patellofemoral arthroplasty. Knee 2008;15:339–47.
13. Leadbetter WB, Seyler TM, Ragland PS, et al. Indications, contraindications, and pitfalls of patellofemoral arthroplasty. J Bone Joint Surg Am 2006;88(Suppl 4): 122–37.
14. Kooijman HJ, Driessen AP, van Horn JR. Long-term results of patellofemoral arthroplasty. A report of 56 arthroplasties with 17 years of follow-up. J Bone Joint Surg Br 2003;85:836–40.
15. Lonner JH, Jasko JG, Booth RE. Revision of a failed patellofemoral arthroplasty to a total knee arthroplasty. J Bone Joint Surg Am 2006;88:2337–42.
16. Leadbetter WB. Patellofemoral arthroplasty in the treatment of patellofemoral arthritis: rationale and outcomes in younger patients. Orthop Clin North Am 2008;39:363–80, vii.
17. Ortiguera CJ, Berry DJ. Patellar fracture after total knee arthroplasty. J Bone Joint Surg Am 2002;84A:532–40.
18. Bengs BC, Scott RD. The effect of patellar thickness on intraoperative knee flexion and patellar tracking in total knee arthroplasty. J Arthroplasty 2006;21: 650–5.
19. Klein GR, Levine BR, Hozack WJ, et al. Return to athletic activity after total hip arthroplasty. Consensus guidelines based on a survey of the Hip Society and American Association of Hip and Knee Surgeons. J Arthroplasty 2007;22:171–5.
20. McGinnis P. Biomechanics of sport and exercise. 3rd edition. Champaign, IL: Human Kinetics; 2013.
21. Engh CA, Collier MB, Hopper RH, et al. Radiographically measured total knee wear is constant and predicts failure. J Arthroplasty 2013;28:1338–44.
22. van Jonbergen HP, Werkman DM, Barnaart LF, et al. Long-term outcomes of patellofemoral arthroplasty. J Arthroplasty 2010;25:1066–71.
23. Robinson EJ, Mulliken BD, Bourne RB, et al. Catastrophic osteolysis in total knee replacement. A report of 17 cases. Clin Orthop Relat Res 1995;(321):98–105.
24. Hendrix MR, Ackroyd CE, Lonner JH. Revision patellofemoral arthroplasty: three- to seven-year follow-up. J Arthroplasty 2008;23:977–83.
25. Ackroyd CE, Newman JH, Evans R, et al. The Avon patellofemoral arthroplasty: five-year survivorship and functional results. J Bone Joint Surg Br 2007;89:310–5.
26. Leadbetter WB, Kolisek FR, Levitt RL, et al. Patellofemoral arthroplasty: a multi-centre study with minimum 2-year follow-up. Int Orthop 2009;33:1597–601.

Rehabilitation of the Patellofemoral Joint

Melody Hrubes, MD, Terry L. Nicola, MD, MS*

KEYWORDS

- Patellofemoral • Treatment • Rehabilitation • Inflammation • Bracing • Therapy

KEY POINTS

- Acute intervention: should commence as soon as the diagnosis of patellofemoral pain syndrome (PFPS) is determined. Initially involves rest, protection, oral or topical medications, or injections, such as corticosteroids, prolotherapy, or platelet-rich plasma. Inflammation and swelling should be addressed with ice, compression, and elevation.
- Subacute phase: once pain and cause of injury have been addressed, correcting all factors that caused PFPS can begin. This is a multifaceted approach and should begin with an in-depth assessment of each individual. Interventions can include therapy, protection through bracing or taping, and foot orthoses if appropriate.
- Therapy: should focus on manual medicine, strength and flexibility, joint proprioception, and stability. Progression through increasingly difficult levels of activity allows the patient to build on skills learned during the previous level.
- Conservative treatment failure: not all cases respond to conservative measures. When a patient is not progressing as expected, multiple reasons should be considered, including chronicity and severity of the symptoms, noncompliance, or undiagnosed medical conditions.

INTRODUCTION TO REHABILITATION APPROACHES FOR PATELLOFEMORAL PAIN SYNDROME

Nonsurgical care by a specialist in physical medicine and rehabilitation is typically a multifaceted approach and can include modalities, bracing, medication, injection, proprioceptive techniques, restoration of normal movement patterns, and overall conditioning. There is evidence that physical therapy interventions have a significant beneficial effect on pain and function compared with no treatment.[1] However, as many as 55% of patients are unsatisfied with their recovery at 3 months, and 40% at 12 months.[2]

Patients are likely to ask about all treatment options, including surgery. A small randomized controlled trial showed that there was no difference in pain or function

Department of Orthopaedic Surgery, UIC Sports Medicine Center, 839 West Roosevelt Avenue, Suite #102, Chicago, IL 60608, USA
* Corresponding author.
E-mail address: tnicola@uic.edu

Clin Sports Med 33 (2014) 553–566
http://dx.doi.org/10.1016/j.csm.2014.03.009
0278-5919/14/$ – see front matter Published by Elsevier Inc.

sportsmed.theclinics.com

between chronic patients with patellofemoral pain syndrome (PFPS) and arthroscopy at 2-year and 5-year follow-up.[3]

GENERAL GOALS

Conservative measures should be attempted for 6 to 12 months before considering surgery,[4] unless there is a specific reason why rehabilitation is unlikely to work (see section on undiagnosed conditions). Goals such as return to sport or work can change throughout the recovery process and must be individualized for greatest chance of success.

CLINICAL OPTIONS FOR REHABILITATION: ACUTE PHASE

The first goal when a patient has been diagnosed with PFPS is to immediately interrupt tissue damage. This interruption can be achieved through rest, decreasing inflammation and swelling, medications (oral, topical or injected), and modalities such as ultrasonography or electrical stimulation.

ACTIVITIES

When addressing rest with your patients, avoidance of pain-inducing activities such as squats, stairs, or uphill running should be discussed. If the patient cannot ambulate without pain, consider making them partial or even non–weight bearing with crutches. Activity modification can be difficult for active individuals, so a practitioner can suggest exercises that do not further damage the patellofemoral joint. These exercises include swimming, pool running, weight lifting seated on bench or ball, or bicycling. In our clinic, we encourage bicycling for comfort, by setting the seat as high as possible to minimize knee flexion at the bottom of the pedal stroke. The patient self-selects the resistance and the revolutions per minute, which allows for pain-free bicycling. We make note of those settings and use them to progress the difficulty of those settings. We consider the elliptical device controversial for patellofemoral rehabilitation, and it should be used with caution, because studies suggest that increased patellofemoral joint contact force occurs during use.[5]

INFLAMMATION AND SWELLING

Inflammation and swelling can be addressed through cryotherapy, compression, and elevation.[6] Cryotherapy may further assist with pain control.[7,8] We recommend applying the ice pack without excessive pressure for 15 to 20 minutes, 2 to 4 times per day, as tolerated. If swelling is present, compression should be used with caution, because it can increase coexisting conditions, such as an inflamed plica or bursitis. In addition, a knee effusion has been found to inhibit the quadriceps muscle.[9] Elevation can reduce the accumulation of interstitial fluid via decrease in hydrostatic pressure. With regard to the lower limb, elevation should be above the level of the pelvis.[6]

MEDICATIONS

Oral and topical medications are available to address pain, which can interfere with activities of daily living and participation in therapy. Studies have shown that naproxen provides significantly better pain relief than placebo in the short-term,[10] but aspirin does not.[11] Oral supplementation, such as glucosamine, has been found to improve pain and function in patients with regular knee pain.[12] Topical diclofenac has also been found to be as effective in improving function and reducing knee osteoarthritis pain as oral nonsteroidal antiinflammatory medications; although systemic absorption must be considered and skin irritation can occur.[13]

MODALITIES

Modalities that could be helpful but have not yet proved effective for PFPS are electrical stimulation and ultrasonography.[14,15] Additional prospective randomized studies are required.

INJECTIONS

Injections have different goals from reducing an inflammatory process (corticosteroids) to inducing a proliferative inflammatory process (prolotherapy or platelet-rich plasma [PRP]).

Typical intra-articular knee joint approaches for injections are the lateral, medial, or infrapatellar approaches.

1. Lateral suprapatellar approach (**Fig. 1**)[16]
   Patient position: supine with knee in extension
   Injection site: at the intersection of lines drawn vertically 1 cm superior to the proximal margin of the patella and horizontally 1 cm below the posterior edge of the patella
2. Medial patellar approach (**Fig. 2**)[17]
   Patient position: supine with knee supported in extension
   Injection site: medial edge of patella, angle needle laterally and slightly upward under patella

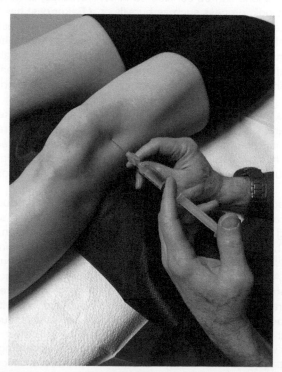

Fig. 1. Injection, lateral suprapatellar approach.

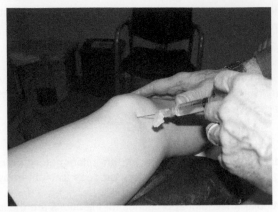

Fig. 2. Injection, medial patellar approach.

3. Infrapatellar approach[16]
   Patient position: supine with affected knee flexed at 30°
   Injection site: 1 cm lateral to the midpoint of the patellar tendon

Corticosteroid injections can provide symptomatic relief but do not address the underlying cause of pathologic patellar tracking. Although they can decrease pain in the short-term when compared with placebo injection, the effect is lost by 4 months.[18] Corticosteroid injections can be considered in severe cases, in which a specific inflammatory pathologic process such as bursitis or a Baker cyst has been identified. Simultaneous anesthetic injection can help address pain and mechanical barriers to therapy participation. It is important to educate the patient that injection therapy is not a 1-time solution. Rather, improved pain control can help to break down physical and mental negative feedback cycles. Thus, it is not a long-term treatment option. A typical solution includes 1 mL steroid solution (40 mg of triamcinolone acetonide) diluted with 8 mL of 1% lidocaine.[16]

Prolotherapy is the process of injecting irritant solutions into weakened or strained ligaments that are a source of pain to induce an inflammatory response, which mimics the normal repair sequence.[19] Solutions classically involved dextrose and lidocaine, which has been found to be effective with intra-articular injection in cases of arthritis.[20] Injured extra-articular structures, such as a tendonosis, can benefit as well.

PRP is prepared from autologous whole blood centrifuged to produce a platelet and plasma concentrate[21] with a high concentration of growth factors,[22] which are essential to stimulating collagen synthesis, mesenchymal cell proliferation, and angiogenesis.[23] Studies have focused more on tendinopathy and less on patellofemoral syndrome as a whole; however, tendinopathy can certainly contribute to the symptoms of PFPS. A recent study in athletes with jumper's knee showed significant pain improvement in the group who received PRP when compared with a group treated with extracorporeal shock wave therapy.[24] However, as with all treatment, PRP should be performed with caution, because adverse events, such as increased pain with patellar tendonitis, have been noted.[25]

Often patients with PFPS have developed trigger points. Identifying these areas for myofascial massage, injecting, or dry-needling can provide an accelerated way to improve tight muscles, such as the iliotibial band (ITB).

CLINICAL OPTIONS FOR REHABILITATION: SUBACUTE PHASE

Once pain and cause of injury have been addressed, correcting all factors that contributed to PFPS can begin. This is a multifaceted approach and should begin with an in-depth assessment of each individual. Interventions can include therapy, protection through bracing or taping, and foot orthoses if appropriate.

Studies have shown that the greatest improvement in pain and function is achieved during the initial 3 months after PFPS diagnosis.[26] Goals must address all modifiable biomechanical factors contributing to pathologic patellar tracking, such as abnormal patellofemoral joint mechanics, altered lower extremity alignment or motion, overtraining, and weak core muscles.[27] Individualized assessment and treatment plans are necessary to optimize therapy, thus maximizing likelihood of success, and should consider all possible contributing factors to the following[1,27]:

1. Patellofemoral realignment: poor patellofemoral tracking can be caused by a tight iliotibial band, decreased patellar mobility, or a weak quadriceps muscle (particularly the vastus medialis obliquus [VMO] mechanism).
2. Correcting kinematic abnormalities: the alignment of proximal and distal joints, and their movement with gait, can also affect patellofemoral tracking. Joints and their movements to consider include subtalar joint pronation, hip internal rotation,[28] or gait deviations, such as knee hyperextension or decreased knee flexion during initial stance. Leg length discrepancy, absolute or relative, has not been found to be a factor in PFPS.[29]
3. Decrease compressive stresses on patellofemoral joint cartilage and overuse: this can be accomplished by introducing relative rest, avoiding increasing activity level too quickly, and ensuring adequate recovery time.

PROTECTION

Protection, with bracing or taping, does not address the underlying biomechanical disease that leads to a patellar tracking problem. However, the idea behind using these interventions for PFPS is to encourage correct patellar tracking, thus limiting further joint damage. Although studies have attempted to show that realignment of the patella through patellar taping and bracing might induce the VMO to fire correctly, there is no evidence to support an improvement in outcome.[30]

BRACING

With regard to bracing, studies have yet to find a difference between pain or functional outcomes between a realignment brace, open patella sleeve, buttress, infrapatellar strap, placebo sleeve, or no brace.[31,32] The goal of the Palumbo dynamic patellar brace (http://www.alimed.com/palumbo-stabilizer-brace.html) is to provide an active, medially displacing force on the lateral border of the patella, maintaining constant pressure during flexion, extension, and rotation of the knee.[32] The Cho-Pat knee strap (http://www.cho-pat.com/products/originalkneestrap.php) functions dynamically as the knee bends and straightens to improve tracking and assist in uniformly distributing pressure over the surface area.[32] The Protonics brace could be set to resist knee flexion in order to increase hamstring activity and inhibit tensor fasciae latae activity.[33] However, it is no longer produced. For a similar effect, we recommend the DonJoy Lateral J knee brace (http://www.betterbraces.com/donjoy-lateral-j-patella-knee-brace). The Special FX knee brace (http://www.burnabyorthopaedic.com/knee-braces/generation/index.php) is a Y-shaped patellar brace to help control patellar movement.[34] The goal of an open patella brace (http://www.alimed.com/alimed-knee-support-with-open-patella.html)

is to guide the patella with an opening to prevent pressing the patella into the femoral condyles. One potential complication of this brace is edema. The Bauerfeind Genutrain brace (http://www.bauerfeindusa.com/en/products/supports-orthoses-knee-hip-thigh/genutrain.html) does not correct patellar tracking patterns,[35] but initial studies reported 50% decrease in pain.[36] In our practice, the clinical usefulness of bracing is limited, particularly in the obese population, because of the loss of surface landmarks to keep the brace in position.

TAPING

Randomized clinical trials have failed to show the benefit of patellar taping over no taping[37] and there is conflicting evidence on the effect of tape on pain and function in the short-term.[31,38] This potential short-term improvement has not been found to last long-term when comparing taping and exercise with exercise alone[31]; however, the short-term benefit to the patient should not be overlooked. The goal of McConnell taping is to achieve a medial shift of patella, centralizing it within the trochlear groove, and thus, improving tracking.[39,40] It has also been shown to inferiorly shift the patella in patients with PFPS.[41]

Kinesiotape has been shown to reduce pain, swelling, and muscle spasm in patients with PFPS. Kinesiotape has been shown to reduce pain and improve quadriceps function for the mechanism of patellar stability in women diagnosed with PFPS.[42] This treatment has not yet been shown to improve the overall outcome of an exercise program.[43]

Although foot orthoses produce earlier and larger improvements in PFPS than flat inserts, studies have yet to show an improvement in physical therapy outcomes.[44] Foot orthoses have been shown to be beneficial for all foot types, not just overpronation, improving both pain and function.[45] Arch type has not been found to be independently associated with PFPS,[46] but a pronated foot posture in relaxed stance has been found in significantly more patients with PFPS when compared with controls.[47–49] Prefabricated orthosis seem to be more beneficial than flat[44]; however, not all patients receiving orthotics benefit from them.[44,45,48] Therefore, it is important to identify the patients most likely to benefit from a prefabricated orthosis. One study found a high likelihood of a patient benefiting from a prefabricated foot orthoses if 3 of the following 4 criteria apply (foot morphology is not a predicting factor):

1. Poor footwear motion control properties (score of <5 on Footwear Assessment Tool)[50]
2. Baseline pain <22 mm (on visual analogue scale)
3. Ankle dorsiflexion range of motion (knee flexed) less than 41.3°[47]
4. Immediate pain reduction during single squat when wearing orthoses[51]

PHYSICAL THERAPY
Manual Medicine

Manual medicine primarily involves mobilization and massage. Mobilization early in PFPS can avoid joint contracture and weakness from deconditioning. A larger patellar tilt angle and larger sulcus angle, and thus, total patellofemoral joint contact area, have been found to be significantly smaller in the PFPS groups compared with the control group.[52] The goal of patellar mobilization is to address these deficiencies. For optimal patellar mobilization, the knee should be in extension or slightly flexed (no more than 20°) (Fig. 3).[27] Myofascial massage can be used to release pathologically tight muscles, specifically the ITB.

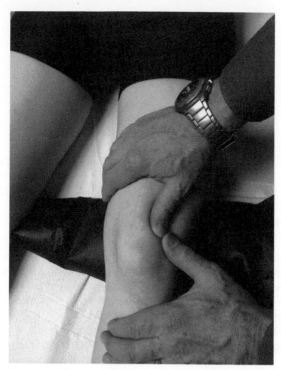

Fig. 3. Manual Medicine: Patellar mobilization.

Strength

Muscle activation involves both strengthening and stretching muscles. Muscles to be strengthened include hip abductors (gluteus medius), hip external rotators, knee extensors, and the core (obliques). Preliminary studies suggest eccentric exercises are more effective than concentric or isometric,[37,53,54] possibly because the primary function of the knee joint is eccentric. Closed chain exercises are preferred over open chain, because there is less full knee extension, and therefore, reduced patellofemoral joint stress.[30] Hip abductors (gluteus medius) have been shown to be weak in PFPS patients compared with controls.[55] The quadriceps, specifically the VMO, promote active medial stabilization of patella within the femoral trochlea,[56] so must be strengthened for optimal performance. However, it is difficult, if not impossible, to isolate the VMO from the rest of the quadriceps muscles, specifically the vastus lateralus muscle.[30] For quadriceps strengthening, we recommend leg press rather than squatting, because the weight can be more easily calibrated for tolerance rather than a person's own body weight. As the patient progresses through simple double-limb exercises, advance to strengthening with single stance to more closely simulate functional gait. This strategy encourages the recruitment of lower abdominal and gluteal muscles for balance during stance phase.[40]

Flexibility

Muscle flexibility is as integral to appropriate patellar tracking as strengthening. It is particularly important to address muscles that are likely to be most arthrogenically inhibited, such as the ITB, hamstrings, and quadriceps muscles.

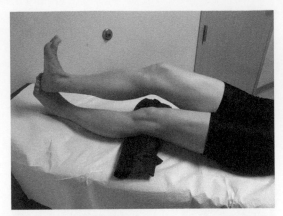

Fig. 4. Flexibility: Knee press with fighting feet.

The act of stretching has been shown to improve muscle relaxation and circulation and reduce soreness.[6] The traditional method of stretching for 30 seconds to 2 minutes is termed static. Patellar mobilization is an example of such stretching. Proprioceptive neuromuscular facilitation (PNF) stretching uses opposing muscles to stretch the target muscle. We use specific exercises using PNF in our clinic, such as knee press with fighting feet (**Fig. 4**) or a hamstring stretch, in which the patient attempts to straighten a raised leg by contracting their quadriceps muscles (**Figs. 5 and 6**).

Stability

Another factor to consider when rehabilitating PFPS is the increased likelihood of finding hypermobile joints in patients with PFPS when compared with controls.[57] Exercises should be designed with this factor in mind. Also, a disturbance of the normal dynamic foot alignment is a risk factor for PFPS development,[58] so the health providers should be watchful, because this could appear as the patient progresses through activity levels. Also, proprioception has been found to be decreased in patients with PFPS with weight-bearing knee flexion at 60% compared with a control

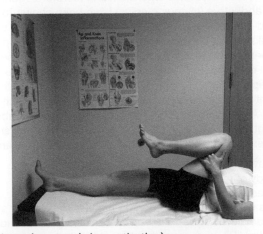

Fig. 5. Flexibility: Hamstring stretch (pre-activation).

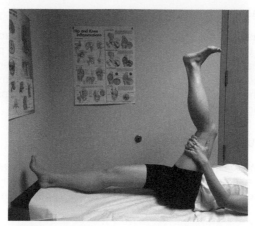

Fig. 6. Flexibility: Hamstring stretch (post-activation).

group.[59] This is another opportunity to address potential avenues for physical therapy failure via focused exercises.

Activity Progression

A patient should not progress to the next level of activity until they are tolerating the current level pain free. Ideally, each stage should be observed by the clinician for early correction of poor gait mechanics, which are likely subconscious to the patient. Throughout the rehabilitation process, the patient should be encouraged to engage in alternative aerobic exercise to preserve baseline cardiovascular fitness and increase the likelihood of activity compliance. This strategy is particularly important, because patients with PFPS have been found to have significantly less muscle endurance when compared with a control group.[29] Activities that we encourage include stationary bicycling and pool running. Once the patient is able to ambulate on level ground without pain, they can progress to uneven ground and stairs.

Once walking on uneven terrain is nonpainful, running can be introduced. Studies have shown that increasing a patient's step rate to 110% of their preferred rate reduces the knee flexion angle and knee extension torque during stance phase. This strategy decreases internal joint loading and leads to a decrease in patellofemoral pain.[60,61] Also, real-time verbal feedback can discourage excessive knee valgus moment, hip internal rotation and adduction, and contralateral pelvic drop during ambulation. There is increasing evidence that individuals can successfully alter their gait mechanics using real-time feedback from an instrumented treadmill.[62,63] This training persisted at 1 month in a small study in women,[31] in which patients attained their baseline training volume and reported pain-free running.

If the patient is successfully running on a treadmill or track, the next step is to start nonlinear movement, such as cutting and turning.

SHOE TYPE

Multiple studies have failed to show effectiveness in recommending a running shoe for arch type.[64] A study of military recruits[65] found the highest injury rate among soldiers who received shoes intended to address foot type. Shoes with too much stability can be harmful to the patient, as well as those with insufficient stability. Also, shoes should be replaced after 643 km (400 miles) or if heel breakdown occurs, and poor fit should not be tolerated.

MAINTENANCE PHASE

Once the patient has progressed through therapy and has achieved their goal activity level without pain, they should be educated on the importance of maintenance to prevent regression and symptom return. They must continue therapeutic exercises at regular intervals to maintain gains. We suggest scheduling a follow-up appointment a few weeks after the patient has been upgraded to full sport to ensure adherence to exercises, stretching, and gait mechanics.

REASONS FOR FAILURE OF CONSERVATIVE TREATMENT

Not all cases respond to conservative measures.[2] When a patient is not progressing as expected, multiple reasons should be considered, including chronicity and severity of the symptoms, noncompliance, or undiagnosed medical conditions.

Symptom Chronicity

It was mentioned earlier that the greatest improvement in patellofemoral pain and function occurs during the initial 3 months.[26] Also, an increased duration of baseline pain (>2 months) has been associated with poor recovery at 3 and 12 months.[2] One review[66] found that 94% of patients continue to experience pain up to 4 years after initial presentation, and 25% reported significant symptoms up to 20 years later.

Pain Severity

Patients with more pain are less likely to successfully treat their PFPS. A higher baseline pain severity, based on the Anterior Knee Pain Scale, was significantly associated with poor recovery.[2] It is possible that pain severity is associated with increased damage to the infrapatellar cartilage. If that damage is severe and irreversible, no amount of protection and rehabilitation can lead to a pain-free existence, and conservative measures are unlikely to be successful.

Noncompliance

When noncompliance is suspected to be to blame for a plateaued or slower than projected improvement, we believe that patient education on PFPS cause and progression can be helpful. Patient noncompliance can occur at any time during their recovery, from initial nonparticipation in therapy or participating in activities that continue to cause pain to discontinuing a home exercise program when symptoms improve. Education can provide the motivational tool required, because the patient participation is essential to their own successful recovery. Consider getting a mental health professional involved, because patients with PFPS were found to have reduced self-perceived health status and increased mental distress when compared with controls.[67]

Undiagnosed Conditions

Patients seldom have a single medical problem. This observation is especially true in a chronic condition such as PFPS. Practitioners should be aware of other medical conditions that share similar symptoms or location of PFPS, because an undiagnosed condition can at best inhibit patient progression, and worst, delay treatment of a life-threatening illness. With the help of previous studies, we have listed other causes of knee pain to assist in creating a differential diagnosis.[1,27]

Lateral pain: lateral retinaculum or ITB friction
Medial pain: medial retinaculum, medial plica, or pes anserine syndrome
Superior pain: quadriceps tendinopathy, suprapatellar bursitis

Inferior pain: patellar tendinopathy, Hoffa's fat pad impingement, or infrapatellar bursitis

Retropatellar pain: articular cartilage damage

Prepatellar pain: prepatellar bursitis

Internal knee derangement: meniscal or ligamentous disease

Diffuse knee pain: pigmented villonodular synovitis, infection, osteoarthritis, or rheumatoid arthritis

Joint line tenderness: meniscal disease or femorotibial osteoarthritis

Ligamentous disease

Referred pain: spine or hip

Tumor

Psychological component of pain

SURGICAL REFERRAL

Some reasons for knee pain should prompt consideration for surgical intervention, because conservative measures are unlikely to be successful. Such diagnoses include angular knee deformity or VMO inhibition caused by knee flexion contracture. Also, any patient with a history of PFPS has an increased risk of later developing patellofemoral osteoarthritis.[68] Thus, if a patient's symptoms change, an additional diagnosis should be considered.

REFERENCES

1. Crossley K, Bennell K, Green S, et al. A systematic review of physical interventions for patellofemoral pain syndrome. Clin J Sport Med 2001;11(2):103–10.
2. Collins N, Bierma-Zeinstra S, Crossley K, et al. Prognostic factors for patellofemoral pain: a multicenter observational analysis. Br J Sports Med 2013;47(4): 227–33.
3. Kettunen J, Harilainen A, Sandelin J, et al. Knee arthroscopy and exercise versus exercise only for chronic patellofemoral pain syndrome: a randomized controlled trial. BMC Med 2007;5:38.
4. Dixit S, DiFiori J, Burton M, et al. Management of patellofemoral pain syndrome. Am Fam Physician 2007;75(2):194–202.
5. Lu T, Chien H, Chen H. Joint loading in the lower extremities during elliptical exercise. Med Sci Sports Exerc 2007;39(9):1651–8.
6. Brukner P, Khan K. Clinical sports medicine. 3rd edition. Sydney (Australia): McGraw-Hill; 2006.
7. Mac Auley D. Ice therapy: how good is the evidence? Int J Sports Med 2001; 22(5):379–84.
8. Basford J. Physical agents. In: O'Connor F, Wilder R, editors. Textbook of running medicine. New York: McGraw-Hill; 2001. p. 535–56.
9. Spencer J, Hayes K, Alexander I. Knee joint effusion and quadriceps reflex inhibition in man. Arch Phys Med Rehabil 1984;65:171–7.
10. Suter E, Herzog W, De Souza K, et al. Inhibition of the quadriceps muscles in patients with anterior knee pain. J Appl Biomech 1998;14(4):360–73.
11. Bentley G, Leslie I, Fischer D. Effect of aspirin treatment on chondromalacia patellae. Ann Rheum Dis 1981;40(1):37–41.
12. Braham R, Dawson B, Goodman C. The effect of glucosamine supplementation on people experiencing regular knee pain. Br J Sports Med 2003;37(1): 45–9.

13. Roth S, Shainhouse Z. Efficacy and safety of a topical diclofenac solution (Pennsaid) in the treatment of primary osteoarthritis of the knee. A randomized, double-blind, vehicle-controlled clinical trial. Arch Intern Med 2004;164(18):2017–23.

14. Werner S, Arvidsson H, Arvidsson I, et al. Electrical stimulation of vastus medialis and stretching of lateral thigh muscles in patients with patello-femoral symptoms. Knee Surg Sports Traumatol Arthrosc 1993;1(2):85–92.

15. Callaghan M, Oldham J. Electric muscle stimulation of the quadriceps in the treatment of patellofemoral pain. Arch Phys Med Rehabil 2004;85(6):956–62.

16. McNabb J. A practical guide to joint & soft tissue injections & aspiration. 2nd edition. Philadelphia: Lippincott Williams & Wilkins; 2010.

17. Saunders S, Longworth S. Injection techniques in orthopaedics and sports medicine. 3rd edition. Edinburgh (United Kingdom): Elsevier; 2006.

18. Arroll B, Goodyear-Smith F. Corticosteroid injections for osteoarthritis of the knee: meta-analysis. BMJ 2004;328(7444):869.

19. Patterson J. An introduction to prolotherapy. In: Anatomy, diagnosis, and treatment of chronic myofascial pain with prolotherapy. Madison (WI): 2001.

20. Banks A. A rationale for prolotherapy. J Orthop Med 1991;13(3):54–9.

21. Mishra A, Woodall J Jr, Vieira A. Treatment of tendon and muscle using platelet-rich plasma. Clin Sports Med 2009;28(1):113–25.

22. Everts P, Knape J, Weibrich G, et al. Platelet rich plasma and platelet gel: a review. J Extra Corpor Technol 2006;38(2):174–87.

23. Sharma P, Maffulli N. Biology of tendon injury: healing, modeling and remodeling. J Musculoskelet Neuronal Interact 2006;6(2):181–90.

24. Vetrano M, Castorina A, Vulpiani M, et al. Platelet-rich plasma versus focused shock waves in the treatment of jumper's knee in athletes. Am J Sports Med 2013;41(4):795–803.

25. Bowman K, Buller B, Middleton K, et al. Progression of patellar tendinitis following treatment with platelet-rich plasma: case reports. Knee Surg Sports Traumatol Arthrosc 2013;21:2035–9.

26. Witvrouw E, Danneels L, Van Tiggelen D, et al. Open versus closed kinetic chain exercises in patellofemoral pain: a 5-year prospective randomized study. Am J Sports Med 2004;32(5):1122–30.

27. Fredericson M, Powers C. Practical management of patellofemoral pain. Clin J Sport Med 2002;12(1):36–8.

28. Souza R, Powers C. Differences in hip kinematics, muscle strength, and muscle activation between subjects with and without patellofemoral pain. J Orthop Sports Phys Ther 2009;39(1):12–9.

29. Duffey M, Martin D, Cannon D, et al. Etiologic factors associated with anterior knee pain in distance runners. Med Sci Sports Exerc 2000;32(11):1825–32.

30. Powers C. Rehabilitation of patellofemoral joint disorders: a critical review. J Orthop Sports Phys Ther 1998;28(5):345–54.

31. Swart N, van Linschoten R, Bierma-Zeinstra S, et al. The additional effect of orthotic devices on exercise therapy for patients with patellofemoral pain syndrome: a systematic review. Br J Sports Med 2012;46(8):570–7.

32. Miller M, Hinkin D, Wisnowski J. The efficacy of orthotics for anterior knee pain in military trainees. Am J Knee Surg 1997;10(1):10–3.

33. Denton J, Willson J, Ballantyne B, et al. The addition of the Protonics brace system to a rehabilitation protocol to address patellofemoral joint syndrome. J Orthop Sports Phys Ther 2005;35(4):210–9.

34. Lun V, Wiley J, Meeuwisse W, et al. Effectiveness of patellar bracing for treatment of patellofemoral pain syndrome. Clin J Sport Med 2005;15(4):235–40.

35. Natri A, Kannus P, Jarvinen M. Which factors predict the long term outcome in chronic patellofemoral pain syndrome? A 7-yr prospective follow-up study. Med Sci Sports Exerc 1998;30(11):1572–7.
36. Powers C, Shellock F, Beering T. Effect of bracing on patellar kinematics in patients with patellofemoral joint pain. Med Sci Sports Exerc 1999;31(12):1714–20.
37. Clark D, Downing N, Mitchell J, et al. Physiotherapy for anterior knee pain: a randomized controlled trial. Ann Rheum Dis 2000;59(9):700–4.
38. Herrington L, Payton C. Effects of corrective taping of the patella on patients with patellofemoral pain. Physiotherapy 1997;83(11):566–72.
39. McConnell J. The management of chondromalacia patellae: a long term solution. Aust J Physiother 1986;32(4):215–33.
40. Greslamer R, McConnell J. The patella: a team approach. Gaithersburg (MD): Aspen; 1998.
41. Derasari A, Brindle T, Alter K, et al. McConnell taping shifts the patella inferiorly in patients with patellofemoral pain: a dynamic magnetic resonance imaging study. Phys Ther 2010;90(3):411–9.
42. Chen P, Hong W, Lin C, et al. Biomechanics effects of kinesio taping for persons with patellofemoral pain syndrome during stair climbing. In: 4th Kuala Lumpur International Conference on Biomedical Engineering. Berlin, Heidelberg (Germany): Springer; 2008. p. 395–7.
43. Adbas E, Atay A, Uiksel I. The effects of additional kinesio taping over exercise in the treatment of patellofemoral pain syndrome. Acta Orthop Traumatol Turc 2011;45(5):335–41.
44. Collins N, Crossley K, Beller E, et al. Foot orthoses and physiotherapy in the treatment of patellofemoral pain syndrome: randomized clinical trial. Br J Sports Med 2009;43(3):169–71.
45. Barton C, Menz H, Crossley K. The immediate effects of foot orthoses on functional performance in individuals with patellofemoral pain syndrome. Br J Sports Med 2011;45(3):193–7.
46. Haim A, Yaniv M, Dekel S, et al. Patellofemoral pain syndrome: validity of clinical and radiological features. Clin Orthop Relat Res 2006;451:223–38.
47. Barton C, Bonanno D, Levinger P, et al. Foot and ankle characteristics in patellofemoral pain syndrome: a case-control and reliability study. J Orthop Sports Phys Ther 2010;40(5):286–96.
48. Sutlive T, Mitchell S, Maxfield S, et al. Identification of individuals with patellofemoral pain whose symptoms improved after a combined program of foot orthosis use and modified activity: a preliminary investigation. Phys Ther 2004;84(1):49–61.
49. Boling M, Padua D, Marshall S, et al. A prospective investigation of biomechanical risk factors for patellofemoral pain syndrome: the Joint Undertaking to Monitor and Prevent ACL Injury (JUMP-ACL) cohort. Am J Sports Med 2009; 37(11):2108–16.
50. Barton C, Bonanno D, Menz H. Development and evaluation of a tool for the assessment of footwear characteristics. J Foot Ankle Res 2009;2:10.
51. Barton C, Menz H, Crossley K. Clinical predictors of foot orthoses efficacy in individuals with patellofemoral pain. Med Sci Sports Exerc 2011;43(9):1602–10.
52. Lankhorst N, Bierma-Zeinstra S, Van Middelkoop M. Factors associated with patellofemoral pan syndrome: a systematic review. Br J Sports Med 2013;47(4): 193–206.
53. Witvrouw E, Lysens R, Bellemans J, et al. Open versus closed kinetic chain exercises for patellofemoral pain. A prospective, randomized study. Am J Sports Med 2000;28(5):687–94.

54. Stiene H, Brosky T, Reinking M, et al. A comparison of closed kinetic chain and isokinetic joint isolation in patients with patellofemoral dysfunction. J Orthop Sports Phys Ther 1996;24(3):136–41.
55. Piva S, Goodnite E, Childs J. Strength around the hip and flexibility of soft tissues in individuals with and without patellofemoral pain syndrome. J Orthop Sports Phys Ther 2005;35(12):793–801.
56. Live F, Perry J. Quadriceps function. An anatomical and mechanical study using amputated limbs. J Bone Joint Surg Am 1968;50(8):1535–48.
57. Al-Rawi Z, Nessan A. Joint hypermobility in patients with chondromalacia patellae. Br J Rheumatol 1997;36(12):1324–7.
58. Thijs Y, Van Tiggelen D, Roosen P, et al. A prospective study on gait-related intrinsic risk factors for patellofemoral pain. Clin J Sport Med 2007;17(6):437–45.
59. Baker V, Bennell K, Stillman B, et al. Abnormal knee joint position sense in individuals with patellofemoral pain syndrome. J Orthop Res 2002;20(2):208–14.
60. Cheung R, Davis I. Landing pattern modification to improve patellofemoral pain in runners: a case series. J Orthop Sports Phys Ther 2011;41(12):914–9.
61. Wille C, Chumanov E, Schubert A, et al. Running step rate modification to reduce anterior knee pain in runners. J Orthop Sports Phys Ther 2013;43(1): A119.
62. Messier S, Cirillo K. Effects of a verbal and visual feedback system on running technique, perceived exertion and running economy in female novice runners. J Sports Sci 1989;7(2):113–26.
63. White S, Lifeso R. Altering asymmetric limb loading after hip arthroplasty using real-time dynamic feedback when walking. Arch Phys Med Rehabil 2005;86(10): 1958–63.
64. Ryan M, Valiant G, McDonald K, et al. The effect of three different levels of footwear stability on pain outcomes in women runners: a randomized control trial. Br J Sports Med 2011;45(9):715–21.
65. Knapik J, Trone D, Swedler D, et al. Injury reduction effectiveness of assigning running shoes based on plantar shape in Marine Corps basic training. Am J Sports Med 2010;38(9):1759–67.
66. Nimon G, Murray D, Sandow M, et al. Natural history of anterior knee pain: a 14-20-year follow-up of nonoperative management. J Pediatr Orthop 1998; 18(1):118–22.
67. Jensen R, Hystad T, Baerheim A. Knee function and pain related to psychological variables in patients with long-term patellofemoral pain syndrome. J Orthop Sports Phys Ther 2005;35(9):594–600.
68. Utting M, Davies G, Newman J. Is anterior knee pain a predisposing factor to patellofemoral osteoarthritis? Knee 2005;12(5):362–5.

Index

Note: Page numbers of article titles are in **boldface** type.

A

Anteromedialization/Fulkerson procedure, advantages and disadvantages of, 524
    surgical technique for, 524–526
Apophysitis, 422, 423
Arthroplasty, patellofemoral, in athlete, **547–552**
      in patellofemoral chondral injuries, outcome of, 491–498
Athlete, anterior knee pain in, **437–459**
    patellofemoral arthroplasty in, **547–552**

B

Bipartite patella, 449
Bursitis, anterior, 432–434
    of knee, 445–446

C

Caton-Deschamps index, 398, 399
Chondrocyte implantation, autologous, in patellofemoral chondral injuries, outcome of,
    489–490
Chondromalacia patellae, 422–423
Chondromalicia patellae, 447–448

F

Foot orthotics, in anterior knee pain, 443

H

Hip muscles, 450
Hyaluronic acid, to stimulate healing, 441–442

I

Iliotibial band syndrome, 446
Infrapatellar fat pad syndrome, 447

J

Joint, zones of loading across, 440

K

Knee, bursitis of, 445–446
    imaging of, 413

Clin Sports Med 33 (2014) 567–572
http://dx.doi.org/10.1016/S0278-5919(14)00046-5
0278-5919/14/$ – see front matter © 2014 Elsevier Inc. All rights reserved.

sportsmed.theclinics.com

Moving?

Make sure your subscription moves with you!

To notify us of your new address, find your **Clinics Account Number** (located on your mailing label above your name), and contact customer service at:

Email: journalscustomerservice-usa@elsevier.com

800-654-2452 (subscribers in the U.S. & Canada)
314-447-8871 (subscribers outside of the U.S. & Canada)

Fax number: 314-447-8029

Elsevier Health Sciences Division
Subscription Customer Service
3251 Riverport Lane
Maryland Heights, MO 63043

*To ensure uninterrupted delivery of your subscription, please notify us at least 4 weeks in advance of move.

Printed and bound by CPI Group (UK) Ltd, Croydon, CR0 4YY

03/10/2024

01040496-0019